Overweight to Fighting Weight

A system to go from morbidly obese to national champion

Written by AJ Watson

OVERWEIGHT TO FIGHTING WEIGHT
A system to go from morbidly obese to national champion

CreateSpace edition. December, 2017.

ISBN 978-1981502547

Written by AJ Watson.

This book is dedicated to my wife Barbara, and my coach and close friend John. Both greatly supported me throughout my journey.

Thanks also go to Paul and Grant for their expert assistance over the years.

Table of Contents

Introduction

My name is Tony and I started this journey at 175kgs.

Today I am 95kgs and hold multiple titles in Brazilian Jiu Jitsu.

This book details how I accomplished that, my mental outlook and changes, my failures and successes. It will show you a way to duplicate this yourself, breaking it into multiple small actions. Depending on where you are on your trek, you may have already accomplished some of the early steps; if so, fantastic. Congratulations on getting that far. This book will help you understand what you have already achieved, and show you how to take it further.

Chances are if you are reading this book then you have struggled with losing weight, or want to see a boost to your motivation in other areas of your life. As someone that has been where you are, and cut a path through the tangled mess that is the weight loss industry, I understand you. This is where my book is different than a lot of others out there. Many programs are great at using weight loss science, but are usually written by people already fit and healthy that have never been more than a few kilos overweight.

They don't understand the mental state many people start with, especially when severely overweight as I was. They have never been fat, never been ridiculed for their obesity. Never avoided pools or the beach because they'd have to take off t-shirts and reveal the true extent of their girth. I am thankful that these health professionals spent time with their research so I could learn. But how could they help address my mental and social issues that contributed to my weight gain, when they couldn't understand them?

A psychologist is needed in many cases. I don't pretend to be one and I've never felt the need to utilise their services. I have known many people that have, and can see the positive impact it made on their lives. I have however researched psychology and as I've lived through it I know a lot about the thought process that goes with obesity. That insight drives many parts of this book.

I am also a certified life coach, a field of study that assists people moving their lives from point A to point B. Even if they are unaware of how to do so, or that point B is even within their reach. Many steps in this book work in unison with the tools and techniques utilised in coaching. They will work without it; though will be greatly enhanced with a life coach by your side.

What I aim to do here is not only show you my meal changes and exercise regime, but also show how my mental state altered. I'll share how I overcame my negative thoughts and barrelled through plateaus.

I gained all of this knowledge through a thirst for understanding. As my wife will attest, I absolutely must know everything even if it doesn't concern me. It's my nature. I can blame and thank my parents for this. As a child I hungered for understanding and often asked questions of how and why. Before long I was asking things they didn't know the answer to. Instead of dismissing it or making something up, my parents instilled in me a simple mantra: look it up.

This was long before the Internet became popular and ubiquitous so all I had was a dictionary, an odd assortment of encyclopaedias and the school library. The skills and knowledge gained were invaluable and formed my love of words and reading.

Overweight to Fighting Weight

The Internet exploded my world and now the guys I train with often refer to me as Google, as I generally have the answer or insight required for the topic at hand.

So when I turned this skill to weight loss my bull-crap detector worked overtime. I tried several diets that I fully understood the science of, but ultimately they failed because they didn't take into account the psychological impact. They also failed to understand the starting point that a lot of overweight people find themselves in.

My meals consisted of mostly eating take-out, snacking on chocolate and washing it down with litres of soft drinks and tubs of ice-cream. You can't instantly go from that to fresh fruit and veggies, healthy snacks and controlled portions. That is why the majority of diets fail and are a waste of your time.

I want to mention right off the bat that this is not a diet book. To me, a diet is a short-term change to reach a desired goal in less than two months. This journey took me nearly a decade and I am still changing things to get better results. It took that long because of all the trial and error, the research required and figuring how to alter the mental conditioning I'd spent nearly three decades building.

I can guide you into doing this far quicker, though I expect it to take years, not months. Lasting change takes time but if you follow the ideas and plans in this book, then you will see some quick results.

I am not a medical professional so I implore you, if you have any conditions or food intolerances then seek their expert advice first. Everything in here works for me, but my body is not the same as yours. I am living proof that the process works, and should work for the majority, however your life is unique and nothing can take everything into account. Even so, everyone can gain some benefit from a lot of these pages.

I'm looking forward to helping you achieve your goals.

A Painted Picture

From the moment I was allowed to make my own decisions, I made poor choices regarding food and exercise. My mother always provided a good home-cooked meal for dinner and a healthy lunch for school with a few snacks and junk food interspersed. I walked everywhere, even taking an hour each way to wander down the street, buy a few packets of basketball trading cards and heading back home. Once I moved out and had to fend for myself, things got a little off track.

Living off the government allowance for students, I had to budget a lot. To even afford to move out of home I shared a house with three friends. Breakfast was easy, cereal and milk in larger portions than my parents allowed because I'm my own man now dammit. Lunch was usually something from the student-discounted-university-cafeteria, like a meat pie and a small bottle of coke. Dinner was ham steaks and two-minute noodles topped with grated cheese. Snacks were chocolate bars or chips. All of this was cheaper than the healthy alternatives. I was doing some martial arts training twice a week but never pushed myself. My weight slowly increased.

Being around 190cm tall with broad shoulders I carry weight well. An extra 10-20kg wasn't that noticeable, but it was enough to slow me down. I had been experiencing back and knee pain for a few years but like any young boy does I ignored it. It became worse through the sporadic martial arts training so I stopped. I figured that it was the training that hurt me, I didn't even think about the extra weight I'd put on as a factor.

Some time passed and my bulk increased. I had zero exercise now that I had a car to get me places. My life consisted of going to classes, doing a part time job and playing video games. I worked at Mars Confectionery as an IT guy, and part of the incentives was samples of their products. Getting a show bag filled to the handle with chocolate every month didn't help my stomach line, especially when it was gone within a week.

Fast forward a few years and things had gotten worse. I was making extra money as a security guard while still attending university. I could now afford more varied food. However my choices over the previous years conditioned me to stay in the same eating habits and thus hamburgers and pizza became my staple. With nothing but fast and junk food, sitting on my butt all day and hobbies that kept me indoors I grew massive. I was at an age where I sought the attention of girls but never found any. This reduced my self-esteem and pushed me further into the corner.

I hated night clubs, my hobbies were what people considered nerdy, my work was solitary and my friends were primarily guys and their girlfriends. I am an introvert and was very shy. I couldn't hold conversations and hate small talk. I could talk for hours about things I enjoyed, but most of them were solo activities that are difficult to enjoy with company. Quite the catch, right ladies?

Part of this was fuelled by my experience in primary and secondary school. I was an outcast. I kept to myself and never did the cool thing everyone else did. I thought it all childish and preferred the company of books, computers or games. I was bullied a lot and didn't fight back because as a larger guy with decent strength I would hurt people and get in trouble for defending myself.

At university I was shocked to find everyone in the class was friendly and genuinely liked me. It was a radical shift and I didn't know how to handle it. My

Overweight to Fighting Weight

formative years were spent mostly alone. I only had two genuine friends until my teens, then I had maybe five. Instead of learning how to speak to people I was bullied. Social events saw me sit quietly in the corner until someone I knew came nearby. So when it came time to be in the real world I was forced to figure out what most people already knew how to do by instinct. Even today dealing with people is a mental struggle and a series of checklists, but I've adapted and thrived.

From this point I only increased in weight. I never thought I was obese however. Yes I knew I was fat but my natural size disguised it well. I could always find an excuse to cover the truth. I wore up to 8XL clothing but I always needed large clothes due to my height. I knew other overweight people that looked obese because they were far shorter than me. By comparison I looked thinner but I was actually far heavier. I played indoor cricket with mates and was exhausted within minutes. I pushed through because I enjoyed it, which is part of where my determination seeded.

Tying my shoelaces caused heavy panting. I assumed I was just unfit rather than understanding my bulk was pushing into my lungs. I needed a special chair to handle my excessive weight but chalked it up to my natural height and bone structure. Walking a block downhill forced me to stop three times to catch my breath while drenching me in sweat. I figured it was just a hot summer day.

I remember attending a course on teaching in the workplace and had to give a presentation. Understanding the material well, I stood up after lunch and led the group in a short round of star jumps to wake them up during their afternoon slump.

Just one minute of that kept me out of breath for the entire 15 minute presentation. I sounded nervous as a result and lost marks as confidence was part of the assessment. I was too embarrassed to admit the truth and let the reduced marks stand.

The single thing that snapped me out of the cycle and made me disgusted with myself was when I went to work for my father to make some extra cash over the holidays. I had been too heavy for the normal bathroom scales for many years so never knew my exact weight. At dad's workplace they had industrial scales with a digital readout. I figured what the hell, I'll weight myself. When it came back as 175.62kg I couldn't get off the scales quick enough. I glanced around ensuring no one had seen the result and continued the day in a funk.

That night I started researching diets.

I had body builder friends so figured they would know how to trim me down with food and exercise. That was a mistake. A body builder's method of training is to eat so that extra mass is available to build muscle. I already had the mass so the training I did used the fuel provided by the food, but did little to reduce the fat already on me.
Yes it helped a little but not the way I envisioned.

I tried low carb diets of all kinds, meal replacement drinks, diets that focused on achieving ketosis and multiple weight loss pills. While I digested the science with enthusiasm, none of it worked. The change was too drastic.
To follow their plan my entire food intake had to change. The expense doubled my food budget and I hated every meal. I lost about 3kg from the attempts but after I quit them the kilos came back on within weeks, usually with a few friends.

When the Wii Fit came out I was excited. Finally I could blend my love of video games and lose weight.

Overweight to Fighting Weight

Further embarrassment resulted when my friends and family saw the TV screaming at me to get off the device as the maximum allowance was 150kg. The advertising failed to mention that little titbit. It actually tried to help by stating the Wii Fit is meant to be used by one person at a time. It was one of the lowest points of my life.

I had to figure out how to shed 20kg just so I could utilise the expensive footrest properly. I knew I had to change my food habits in a way that wasn't diametrically opposed to my current condition. I had a limited understanding of goal setting back then but knew enough to realise it had to be done in small steps.

That is when things started to change for the better.

<u>Meal Alterations</u>

People react poorly when told to stop doing something, even if it's in their best interest. Removing something brings a negative mindset, where adding something is generally seen as positive.

To tap into this the first thing is not actually removing any food but to add something else in. So today, after you put this book down and are preparing your dinner, add in a serve of fresh vegetables. Preferably this will be green veggies such as broccoli but any will suffice for now. A good serve would be two cups.

Add this in to every meal this week and ensure the veggies are the first thing you eat on the plate. You can leave other parts of the meal uneaten if you get full, though you probably won't assuming you are like me. If you are getting takeout grab a pack of instant veggie bags from the frozen supermarket section on your way home. They are a good serve and can be cooked in a microwave in a few minutes.

This will establish a few baselines for you. First, the veggies will begin to fill you so you may find you can't finish the rest of the meal. Considering that meal is likely junk that is a good thing. If you dislike veggies it will help with actually eating them. Consuming the hated food first you can "wash away" the taste with your normal meal. I despised veggies as all my tastebuds had access to for decades was sugar and junk.

Veggies were bland and tasteless, why would I want to eat them? Doing it this way helps break down your psychological issues for eating healthy. I don't pretend to know what brought you to this point but there are some commonalities with dealing with the issues. This process won't solve all your emotional struggles but will go some way towards improving them.

Second, it will begin planting a habit. You will be spending a lot of weeks altering your meals so they differ from the week before. This process establishes the framework to do so.

Third, it builds the basis of learning how to set goals. Stating the above task as a useful goal would look something like this:

Every day this week I will add a 2 cup serve of vegetables to my dinner and ensure I eat it first.

You can see how this is specific, has a time frame and can be measured. That is critical to setting goals which is something I'll cover in more depth later in this book. For now we'll continue with what the next few months will look like.

You spend a week eating an extra serve of veggies with meals and may notice a slight weight change, mood improvements, increased energy levels or simply more regularity. If you don't that's fine but you should expect it shortly. The next step is to replace some takeaway meals with a home cooked meal. This could be as simple as meat and two veg, a microwave meal or oven baked chips and crumbed chicken-breast steak. Each home cooked meal should have a serve of veggies.

Doing this starts to build the habit of preparing your own meals. This is crucial in future steps so we know exactly what is going into our food. Normally the best meal to replace is dinner however a prepared sandwich lunch is also great. Just ensure to include leafy greens such as spinach and lettuce in the mix.

You might be seeing a pattern here. We are not removing poor food choices in a massive leap, but are replacing some of it with good healthy choices while still enjoying the junk food. The aim over the first few months is to retrain your brain to reach for a healthier alternative instead of relying on the same old junk.

To aid in this, visualise what eating healthy looks like. Everyone, at the core, knows what food is healthy and what food is crap. There are several grey areas but mostly you can tell just by looking at it. A burger dripping with oil may be tasty, but it is clearly an unhealthy choice. Close your eyes and go to a time in the future, say one month from now, and see yourself eating a healthy meal, consuming healthy snacks and drinking tasty and healthy liquids.
Can you see it?

This is what you are working towards. By the time we are done you will have gained the skill to choose the healthy alternatives but still eat a chocolate bar or pizza every now and then. By the end of the first few months the goal is to only eat takeout once a week and have a few unhealthy snacks a day. Those of you reading this that are only looking to drop 15 to 20kg may think that is still high. But if you are in the position I was, of needing to drop well over 50kg then this level is likely a radical reduction.

Step 1 - The 8 Week Guide to Retrain your Brain

Before we move on I want to spell out what you could do for the next few months in little steps. It is important to keep each step small. I began my journey with eating takeout every meal, having a packet of chocolate bars, a bag of chips, a couple litres of Coke and a bowl of ice-cream each day. You cannot immediately change that to home-cooked meals, two or three chocolate bars and a can of coke each day. If you tried that now you would fail within days. I know because I attempted exactly that, and more extreme changes. I sought to change overnight and failed miserably.

So the key is small steps to make gradual changes. It helps to add reminders into your phone so you are alerted at the appropriate times. This is a great start:

Week 1

- I will take a "before" photo of myself, note down my pants, top and bra sizes and my weight. I will measure my waist, hips and neck circumferences. I will use this to calculate my body fat percentage, and keep these in a safe place for reference later. (Repeat this step every four weeks only)
- Every day this week I will add a 2 cup serve of vegetables to my dinner and ensure I eat it first.
- Every morning I will visualise what eating perfectly healthy looks like.
- Every day I will park my car in the furthest spot from my destination allowing me to walk a greater distance.

Week 2

- Three days this week I will prepare a home-cooked meal instead of takeout and ensure it includes a 2 cup serve of vegetables which I will eat first.
- I will smile at myself in the mirror every morning with genuine mirth.
- Three times this week I will walk to the furthest corner of my neighbourhood block and back again.
- I will continue with all previous week's steps

Week 3

- Every day this week I will prepare at least one meal from home, ensuring it includes a 2 cup serve of veggies which I will eat first.
- Every time I greet people I will flash them a genuine smile.
- Three times this week I will walk around my entire block.
- I will continue with all previous week's steps

Week 4

- Every day this week as soon as I wake up I will drink 500ml of water.
- Every day this week I will eat at least one serve of fruit as a snack.
- Every day this week I will walk around my entire block.
- I will continue with all previous week's steps

Week 5

- Every day this week I will drink a large glass of water or coconut water with my dinner.
- Every day this week I will eat two serves of fruit as a snack.
- Every time this week when someone asks "How are you?" I will reply with an enthusiastic "I'm great" or "I'm fantastic".
- I will continue with all previous week's steps

Overweight to Fighting Weight

Week 6

- Every day this week I will drink a large glass of water or coconut water with my lunch and dinner.
- Three days this week I will prepare every meal from home, ensuring it includes a 2 cup serve of veggies which I will eat first.
- Every day this week, immediately after getting out of bed I will do at least three push ups.
- I will continue with all previous week's steps

Week 7

- Five days this week I will prepare every meal from home, ensuring it includes a 2 cup serve of veggies which I will eat first.
- Every day this week, after getting out of bed I will do at least five push ups and five crunches.
- At least once this week, I will ask a service person (eg supermarket cashier) how their day has been and I will listen to their reply. I will share something about my day with them. I will give them a sincere compliment and warm smile.
- I will continue with all previous week's steps

Week 8

- At least three times this week I will eat a handful of unsalted, unroasted nuts as a snack. (If you have a nut allergy, increase your fruit serves)
- This week I will eat at least two types of fruit or vegetables I have not had before.
- Every day this week, after getting out of bed I will do at least ten push ups and ten crunches.
- I will continue with all previous week's steps

Ensure each week you are adding to the steps for all previous weeks. So in week 5 you will be doing all steps from week 1 through to week 5.

You probably noticed there are a few non-food related things added in there. I will explain them further in the following pages. They have more to do with your mindset and exercise, which are both vitally important if you intend to succeed.

Notice I have not mentioned to stop eating junk food or drinking sugary beverages. Your willpower won't allow you to stop that at this point. What the above will do is train you to make better choices with your meals, and make you fuller so you should snack less. Even if you haven't lost much weight over this time, you will be healthier and should feel better in yourself. The significant weight loss is coming but first we need to understand the finer points of food intake so we can make a powerful change in the following months.

Understanding Nutrition

Thus far all we have done is altered how we are eating based on our inner knowledge of what is healthy and what isn't. Where we will see the best results is by understanding the nutrition and ingredient information on food packages. This is part of The Energy Budget step in the Next Steps chapter below but we need a good understanding as soon as possible to begin adjusting our mentality.

There are a lot of misconceptions when it comes to food. Things that seem good for us one day are found to be bad the next. Just because it's "natural" doesn't mean it is good for us. Arsenic is natural but you wouldn't sprinkle it on your cereal. Some processed foods can be of great benefit. Genetically modified doesn't mean it's worse, for example all bananas from the grocer (Cavendish variety) are identical genetic clones. Most foods have been modified by man before it hits the supermarket isle, even "natural" ones.

With so much misinformation and aggressive sales tactics the lines are blurred and we can't trust any flashy slogans or banners on the package. We instead need to focus on the fine print of ingredients and nutrition details.

This will not be an in depth scientific analysis of micro nutrients as we don't need that level of detail. What we need is the knowledge of how to interpret what food manufacturers place on their packages by law, and what that means for making healthy choices.

Ingredients

Ingredients are listed in order of their percentage of the total product, so the first few are what the food or drink mainly consist of. This is why many companies use multiple sources of sugar. That way they can break it down on the label. If it stated 40% sugar people would leave it alone. Compare that to 12% fruit juice concentrate, 10% maltose, 8% corn syrup, 6% sucrose, and 4% dextrose. It aims to confuse the consumer. We won't fall for their tricks any longer.

We are looking for foods that contain ingredients mainly from words we understand as food, such as whole grains, vegetables, fruit, various meats etc. Ensure they take up the bulk of the list. Always treat all sugar sources (refer below) as one lumped sum instead of individual items.

When seeking food with grains ensure they are whole grains. With the word "whole" missing you can be assured that there has been some processing and you are likely only getting part of the grain. This is generally the part with minimal nutrients. Manufacturers proudly state they use whole grains and it is usually the first or second ingredient on the list.

Extracts or concentrate are a poor substitute for the real thing, but is easier to increase profit margins. Pay attention to the type of oil used (if any). Some of the better oils are olive, flaxseed, sunflower and avocado. The main thing to avoid here are partially-hydrogenated fats and shortening.

Ensure the characteristic ingredient is prominent. Raspberries in raspberry jam are a good example. While raspberries may not be the primary ingredient by weight, they must be in the list and are usually in the first few.

Nutrition Information

This is where most people look first, but we will do this second after the ingredients have passed muster.

Overweight to Fighting Weight

The main things concerning us are:
1. Energy in kilojoules (kj)
2. Protein in grams (g)
3. Fat in grams (g)
4. Carbohydrates in grams (g)
5. Sugars in grams (g)
6. Fibre in grams (g)
7. Sodium in milligrams (mg)

Energy

This is basically a numeric representation of how much fuel the food or beverage adds to your tank. It doesn't care what makes up the fuel just that it is there to use. Using energy to track our daily intake makes it easy to see where we can improve.

To illustrate, about 250ml of Coke is 450kj where the same quantity of coconut water is 200kj. So you can have over 500ml of coconut water to match the energy of half as much Coke. This will quench your thirst, make you fuller, add far more nutrients and introduces a hell of a lot less sugar.

My current daily energy intake, taking into account my age, sex, activity levels, current and goal weights is between 8500kj and 12500kj. The exact number is up to trial an error and requires checking your weight at weekly intervals. If you increase weight in the week then drop 500kj a day for the next week and try again. I suggest starting in the middle of the range to begin. There are thousands of websites and phone apps that calculate this for you, though my favourite is www.8700.com.au (check the link for "your ideal figure").

The key here is to look at the numbers of what you are thinking of eating and make an informed choice. That mouth-watering hamburger with 3500kj is at least a third of your daily budget. Do you want to use that much on a single food item? This doesn't include the hot chips and soft-drink that generally comes with the burger as a meal. Some pizzas will be more than your entire daily allotment, so you can only afford a slice or two if you intend to eat more than once a day. This takes practice and is why we don't do it all at once.

Protein

The main two functions of proteins (they have more uses than these though) are to build and repair body tissue, and to provide energy. The main energy source is from carbs, though the energy from proteins is a good boost but most importantly makes you feel satiated for longer. If you feel fuller for longer, then you are less likely to reach for a snack. Protein is a good thing but too much can cause health issues, and may cause gas. As a general guide, consume 1g of protein a day per kilogram of your weight.

Eggs, fish, pork, chicken, beans and yoghurt are all great protein sources so should be included in meals. Assuming you are starting where I did, I am taking a leap that you are not vegan. But to ensure a more complete book there are vegan choices here. While I personally don't recommend a strict vegan diet, you can still get protein from things like green peas, quinoa, raw nuts, sunflower seeds and tofu.

The main thing for our protein purposes at the early stages is to feel satiated. Only consuming the vegan choice will mean eating a lot more green peas to feel the same level of fullness as eating some chicken breast. Protein powder is another great choice which can be easily added to a breakfast smoothie.

Overweight to Fighting Weight

Fat

Our bodies require fat. It is the backup fuel source after carbs. Fat helps our body absorb vitamins and is insulation for our core temperature. The problem is that fat has double the amount of energy per gram as carbs and protein. You should limit your fat intake to between 20% and 35% of your daily energy. As 1g of fat has around 37kj we can easily calculate our daily maximum. For me that would be between 55g and 100g of fat per day. A Snickers bar has 12g of fat (and over 1000kj) so that simple snack is a good chunk of our daily allotment. Having that means we will have a harder time fitting the rest of the day's meals into the budget.

We have another pattern emerging here. If we can see exactly how much the junk food is adding to our daily maximum intake, we can start to see they are not worth it.

I remember a time in the early days when I was still figuring this entire thing out. I had a Snickers and a can of Coke around lunch time. I thought it won't hurt; I won't eat much for the rest of the day. But because I wasn't satiated and I was still thirsty I keep reaching for small snacks; a handful of nuts here, a glass of coconut water there. By dinner I had maybe 100kj left of my daily budget. If I didn't have the Coke and Snickers I would have had and extra 1500kj. But I did consume them so my choice was to go over budget, or not eat dinner while my stomach was growling up a storm.

This is where the struggle kicks in. It takes willpower to overcome this, which is a finite resource. I'll delve into that later but we need to acknowledge this process is slow. Failure in one day does not mean failure overall. I've failed more times than I can count. The trick is to keep going and remember why you are doing this.

Carbohydrates

Carbs have gotten a bad reputation in diet circles thanks to the "low carb diet" being heavily promoted. I've tried low and no carb diets and failed in under a week to maintain it. Carbs are the primary body fuel source but are also needed for proper brain function and organ operation. Denying your body of carbs means it doesn't have what it needs when it needs it. Carbs are essential for digestive health and waste removal, i.e. poop. No one likes being constipated but that is what a no carb diet will send you towards.

You should have between 45% and 65% of your daily energy from carbs, but we have to pick the right ones. Carbs come in simple and complex forms. Simple is basically your sugars, whether added via processing or natural sugars such as in fruit. Complex carbs are starches and come from whole grains, legumes and certain vegetables such as potatoes. The majority of complex carbs also contain fibre which increases satiety.

For our purposes we want to reduce added sugar and processed grains. Aim for carbs with whole grains rather than refined. You can determine this by a glance at the ingredients on the package. As previously mentioned, the word "whole grain" is usually in the first two ingredients of appropriate food. If it is missing you can practically guarantee the grains have been refined and the goodness extracted to the bin.

Sugars

Closely related to carbs, the sugars are actually a subset on the label. We want to limit the amount of sugars and there is a very simple guide for this. Compare the carbs value with the sugars. If they are the same, put

Overweight to Fighting Weight

it back on the shelf. This means the only carbs you will get here is sugar.

Also look at the amount of sugar per 100g. If it's fewer than 4g then it's a good choice. Otherwise look elsewhere for your carb needs.

Some sugar is essential so don't remove it entirely. We need roughly 5% of our energy intake as sugar. What we want however are natural sugars not added ones. Again the ingredients list will help with that. Practically anything ending in "ose" is a sugar. Fructose, dextrose, glucose, maltose, sucrose etc are all added sugar. Companies also like disguising added sugar as fruit juice concentrate, corn syrup or invert sugar just to confuse the consumer.

The more of these terms on the label, the more percentage is added sugar. Leave them alone and grab something else.

Fibre

Most people know fibre is useful for regular bowel movement but it is also the main ingredient to make us feel full. If we are full we generally don't want to eat more so we can limit our weight gain. The higher the fibre the less likely we are to eat more. Notice I said "less likely" not "guaranteed not to".

Part of the reason I put on so much weight is that I didn't want to miss out on any "good" food. This was things like sweets, roast potatoes, savoury treats and the gamut of snacks. Even though I was full, I always had room for apple crumble with custard and ice-cream topped with chocolate sprinkles. Today I still receive the urge to eat more when I'm full just because someone brought out a new treat to share.

Saying no uses up more of our finite willpower, which I promise we'll get to soon. We can plan for the dessert by eating less of the actual meal, but that is defeating the purpose of making the right food choices.

If you are really struggling with this, a certified life coach can help alter your habits that no longer serve you. Turning something you like such as chocolate into something you dislike can be achieved in a single session. My contact details are at the end of this book. I can assist either in person or over the phone.

Plant based foods have fibre which is why I've been getting you to add leafy greens and vegetables to your meals. Also include whole grains, air popped corn (no butter or oil added), carrots, cucumbers, raisins, grapes and tomatoes to name but a few.

On the packet, look for foods with over 2.5g of fibre. A great source would have more than 5g per serve.

Women need around 25g per day and men need about 38g. Exceeding that will impact your poop but can be balanced with low fibre foods such as chicken. Assuming you are getting far less than that due to your existing eating habits, you will need to start slow.

Add in an extra 2g to 5g per day and see how it affects your mood and digestion. If no issues then add in a further 2g to 5g each day until you reach the above. You will also need to increase your water consumption, and watch out for increased flatulence. If you are too gassy then lessen the fibre intake tomorrow and drink another glass of water.

Not all labels will show fibre, if it is absent generally that food or drink doesn't contain any.

Sodium

This is required to maintain blood pressure, and too much will put you at higher risk of high blood pressure and stroke. The average amount per day should be around 1500mg with a maximum of 2300mg. If you are over 50 then drop that average a couple hundred. Unless you doctor tells you otherwise.

Pre-packaged microwave meals, smoked lunch meats, packet mixes, garlic salt, processed cheese and creamed vegetables are examples of food with high sodium content. That doesn't mean they are bad, they should simply be limited.

For low sodium choices we can grab fresh meat, fish and poultry, block cheeses, fresh or frozen vegetables, garlic powder or homemade versions of packet mixes.

Not all labels will show sodium, if it is absent generally that item doesn't contain any or the amounts are miniscule.

Serves

The final part of this is to understand serving sizes. Most labels include serves per 100g, however that is not a suitable reference for snacks. Manufacturers like to trick you into saying their product has 2 serves when the vast majority of people consume the lot in one sitting. Chocolate bars often fall into this category.

Ensure you check the serving suggestion at the top of the nutritional information section. You can then multiply the values by the number of serves you expect to consume.

Keep in mind a lot of these are average figures that are rounded down. Companies like to put their product in the best possible light. So while the package may say there is 1g of fat per serve, the reality may increase that figure if you have 6 serves, giving you 1.2g per serve and thus 7.2g instead of the 6g you assumed. The 100g column and some math can help discern this. Divide the 100g by the serving suggestion size, for ease I'll assume

25g and thus one quarter. Multiply the 25g value for fat by 4 and compare to the 100g value. Assuming the 100g value is higher, the lower value has been rounded down. You phone calculator can help greatly when in the supermarket.

When calculating values round up to the nearest 0.5g. Other than saving your sanity, overestimation is better than being underdone. The rounding won't impact your totals much, but it gives you some headroom.

What to do with all this

With this understanding we can make informed choices of the food we buy. We can still eat poor health choices, but in moderation. Always weigh up the food or drink item with how much of your daily energy it will consume.

I want to clarify here that you will not be doing this tracking for the rest of your life. We need this in the initial stages to understand how to make great heathy choices. Each person will reach the tipping point at a different pace. Expect to count energy and nutrients for 6 to 18 months. At that point all you'll need to do is look at the ingredients and nutrition panel of unfamiliar food and add it in if appropriate.

Part of the mental issues with food arises with how we associate it to emotions. Likely you tie eating junk food with negative emotions and a healthier choice with positive ones. If you have a can of Coke you might feel disappointed in yourself and guilty.

The problem with this is the constant mental assault of feeling unhappy and angry. If you eat a poor food choice simply acknowledge it and move on. A simple acknowledgment might be to mentally state "I deserve better than this."

Overweight to Fighting Weight

There are minimal negative emotions with that thought and it provides a small mantra to tap into. Eventually you will believe you deserve better which does wonders for breaking bad habits.

Another method that worked well for me was to really think about how I physically and emotionally felt when consuming an item. As I've mentioned a few times, I drank a lot of Coke. When I gazed inward I noticed my thirst wasn't quenched. My mouth was dry. I felt guilty at having it when water was free and two steps further away. I now needed to exercise harder and restrict other food intake to balance it out, which angered me as I was going so well all day before hand. Having a can of Coke is now associated with guilt and anger.

So what happens when I have another can of Coke? The anger and guilt spirals in out of habit. Why would I want to feel that? Now I understood everything that was happening to me I could change it. Altering the thoughts with the example mantra above allows the negativity to bugger off and leave me to more pleasant emotions.

This all ties in with willpower, as you will see later. A life coach can assist greatly with improving your self-talk as well. For now we'll move into something a bit more physical.

Exercise and Plateaus

While we can start exercising from day one, it can be overwhelming to work on our food habits and exercise all at once. I recommend doing the first 2 months as shown in the Meal Alterations chapter. This eases us into the changes and includes some basic exercise which will get us prepared for the next step.

If you find it too easy then skip ahead a week but still combine everything. For example if you are at week 3 and find it too easy, next week add week 4 and week 5 together and treat that as your week 4. This process needs to take at least a month to aid in forming new good habits, and small steps are best to gain momentum.

There are some exercise routines later in this book to get you started, however I believe everyone should have a physical hobby such as a sport. It gets us moving, provides another reason to lose weight and get healthy, but mainly keeps us motivated. A good hobby will have different levels of fitness and strength that we can strive towards. The more minor goals we can add in, the easier it becomes to cross them off. That isn't to say we should have easy goals, just focus on a smaller subset of the task.

As you might expect from the book cover, my chosen activity is martial arts. When I was still dropping weight, I was around 130kg from memory; I struggled to perform some specific techniques. The position involved in the grapple was very controlling, however I had to rely on strength instead of technique to maintain it, and put my arm in jeopardy of hyperextension from myself.

My goal was to perform this technique without hurting myself. I could have set goals to practice it over and over until I got it right but with a simple review it became clear every trouble I had was due to my lack of flexibility.

Overweight to Fighting Weight

I could have worked on overall flexibility but that would take longer to get my core achievement of performing the move and not holding up my training partners. So I set my goal to gain the flexibility for this specific move by the start of the session next week. Each day I only stretched the specific region needed for that technique, and did so for less than 15 minutes per day including the time it took to warm up.

By the end of the week the technique was easy, I had greater control and was able to move forward. That minor goal on one key aspect was my primary focus. Sure it was hard but breaking it into daily tasks didn't make it seem overwhelming.

These little stepping goals also help with plateaus in one area. When weight loss slows or motivation wanes, we can focus on our sport specific goals. When sports goals begin to plateau the weight loss goals are there to work on again. We switch focus to avoid dips in motivation and to give us a break.

When I think of a plateau I think of all the times I couldn't be bothered losing weight anymore. It had been years and while I made some progress I really wanted to eat more pizza and chocolate. As I mentioned, it's insanely difficult to stop eating the food that brought you to your excessive weight. You are fighting habits established and reinforced over decades. My default setting when feeling low is to splurge and eat junk. When I want a snack at times of stress, often my first thought is to grab some chips or chocolate. What stops me most of the time is the thought of breaking my goals, or how much extra work I'll need if I eat junk. Don't get me wrong, I still enjoy junk food, but in moderation.

Now this determination took me years to cultivate. I fought tooth and nail to do this myself, though you have an advantage. This book will guide you into doing it yourself a bit later, but if you struggle contact me so we can work together and smash down barriers.

Before we can get to all that I need to iterate something now:

We can't stop plateaus.

No one can remain 100% focussed and motivated for years or even months. We will run out of steam. Work and family will consume time and energy we intended to spend on ourselves. It will get too much for us at times and we need to take a break. This is natural and I couldn't have continued without having rests along the way.

I can instantly tell when I reach a plateau as my food intake degrades into old patterns. Recognition is the key to tackling these. The moment I see the degradation I make a new broad goal. I set an upper limit to my weight and won't allow myself to go over that.

Last year I was 107kg and was tired of competing in that weight bracket. The reason for this is in Brazilian Jiu Jitsu, and most other combat competitions, the upper limit is 97kg. Anything over that was lumped into a single bracket. So while the lower divisions enjoy no more than 6kg difference, I often faced people with over 30kg of weight advantage. At nearly 40 with chronic back and knee issues (mostly because of my previously excessive weight) my body can't handle that anymore.

So my goal was to compete in the 92 to 97kg bracket. With that set I went about planning my reduction. Unluckily for me, when I was about to start I sprained a ligament in my back. I couldn't train due to excessive pain for weeks. It took 2 months to be ready to train properly, but the flu had other ideas which knocked me out for another couple weeks. So what started as ample time to drop weight, turned into a rushed 9 weeks. I can tell you it sucked.

Rapid weight loss is not recommended, in fact half a kilo a week is considered safe for a healthy person to ensure it stays off. I had to lose almost three times that. So with the help of coaches and medical staff I was able to create a plan. My food intake was heavily restricted; I had to step up exercise while maintaining normal training sessions. It was the worst 2 months of my journey but I learned a lot, most of which I share in this book. I would go back and do it again just to gain the insights from it.

I reached my goal early and actually dropped to 92kg, but there was a setback. There was no one to compete with in my age, weight and skill level at that competition. My choices were to go up in weight category, which I strived so hard to avoid, or go down in age group. I wanted my work to pay off so dropped in age, giving away 15+ years to my opponents. People under 30 don't realise just how much your conditioning and recovery drops as you age. This is why we don't see many professional athletes older than 35. Sure there are some exceptions but their careers definitely wind down. It takes longer to recover from injury and we can't keep up the intensity of the younger athletes.

As a result of all this, I went harder than normal and eventually got injured. It's part of martial arts competition that eventually you will be injured in some manner. We have ways to deal with it, which helped teach me to train how I can, not how I want to.

The culmination of all this is that my motivation waned because my goals were now superfluous. I wanted to compete in multiple tournaments but couldn't due to the injury. So my effort in eating right slipped. I always planned on having a pizza and Coke, with ice-cream for desert as a reward after the comp. I still had that but as my training levels had to drop off to cater to the injury I put on some weight. I was able to maintain a weight of around 94kg for a month until the junk food piled up piece by piece. This was my new plateau.

So I set a target. I would not allow myself to go higher than 100kg. When that happened I had to get under 97kg before I was allowed junk food again. This way I could fight the plateau in miniscule steps. It took me a couple weeks to put the weight on, and a week to take it back down.

This does fly in the face of what I mentioned earlier of half a kilo a week being safe. This is because I've been on this journey for years and my body is at a state primed for dropping weight. I have around 15-20% body fat which is in the ideal to athlete brackets. Just by removing the extra junk for a week I'll drop the kilos. Many athletes enjoy this ability but it can be abused. You shouldn't compete in a weight category more than 5kg lighter than you walk around at. Some fighters drop 20kg to compete, usually in two to three months but that is too extreme and very hard on your body and organs.

I've built the ability to slip up for a day or two while dropping weight so it isn't onerous. Weight always fluctuates by a few kilos, even over the course of a day. This is normal so don't fall into the trap of weighing yourself more than once a day. The best time to weigh yourself is in the morning directly after any bowel movements and before breakfast. This removes as many variables as possible. While I weigh myself daily, I am using this as data points in my self-experimentation. Generally you only want to weigh yourself once a week.

With my tools assembled, I have maintained equilibrium for about 8 months. I don't feel quite ready to be overly strict with diet again but am stepping up training. The extra exercise will help me drop weight without having to alter the diet.

Overweight to Fighting Weight

This way by the time I'm ready to compete again, I'll only need to shed a few kilos to be between 91kg and 95kg.

Because I have the tools and knowledge to drop weight safely I know this won't be an issue. These same tools are explained in this book.

The take away from this is that when you recognise you are at a plateau, set an upper limit of weight gain and when you reach that level, work the system to come back down. When you are mentally ready to continue in force, it will be that much easier to drop. On average I found I lost motivation every 15 to 20kg dropped, so allowed an upper limit of 5kg to 10kg of weight gain. Every time I stuck with that I dropped over 25kg before the next plateau. If I didn't stick to the upper limit my next motivation took longer to find and I shed no more than 15kg.

Once you hit the wall you need to understand why you did. For me in the most recent wall it was the injury from comp and how I let it affect my attitude. Because I understood the motivational damage I could combat it. My goals can then be reworked to fix that, breaking large issues into manageable chunks to get back on track.

When you reach a plateau take the photos and measurements from week one again for comparison. This is extremely useful as it shows you just how far you have come already. This provides motivation to keep going. I'd also recommend sharing these before and after pictures with your family and friends. They can see the progress you made and the kudos they will send your way is also a great motivator to continue the journey. Facebook is great for this as you control who can see it, and next year it will remind you of the post for a great look back at how far you have come.

Part of restoring my motivation is to keep up with my martial arts successes. If I put on weight it will negatively influence my training. When you shed even 5kg your performance increases dramatically. That is a powerful motivator and can keep you on track. Having this reason to lose weight outside of general health is critical. If I only had health as a reason to drop the fat I likely would've stopped at about 130kg.

Multiple motivational avenues work off each other to keep you going. One of the biggest additional motivators I had recently was to start a blog detailing several concepts included in this book. Even if I didn't have a massive captive audience, I still had enough people look at it to keep me in check. I made posts stating my short term goals and documented each step of the way. I felt the drive to actually make it work as I didn't want to face the disappointment from my audience. It helped that they were family, friends and training partners meaning I'd be seeing them every day. The thought of seeing their judgment, imagined or otherwise, was enough motivation to ensure I succeeded. You can use blogspot to create a free blog for this purpose linked to your google account (we all have one of those right?).

This is why it's important to have a physical hobby. The drive you receive from others is more valuable than diamonds. I wouldn't be where I am today if it wasn't for my coach and great friend John, his belief in me and his unwavering support.

Outside that support, martial arts is an outlet for my daily frustrations. If work or daily events get me down or angry, a few minutes on the mat washes those feelings away. I may take it out on an inanimate punching bag, or get so swept up in the technique that making it flawless is all I can think about. If you want to de-stress then martial arts is perfection.

Overweight to Fighting Weight

When I was young my father introduced me to Chuck Norris movies. I instantly fell in love with the martial arts and absorbed all I could. My teachers growing up were Chuck Norris, Bruce Lee, Jackie Chan, Richard Norton, Cynthia Rothrock, Jean-Claude Van Damme, Mark Dacascos, Don 'The Dragon' Wilson, Bolo Yeung and a plethora of others. I wanted to be like them, not as an actor but as someone that dedicated their life to perfecting an art form. I've had the great fortune of actually meeting and training with some of them as well.

Having this connection to a childhood dream made it easy to choose my physical hobby when the time came. If you don't have one then I suggest following my footsteps as the health benefits are incredible. Here are just a few:

- Heightened knowledge of how your body feels
- Perform feats that are thought too difficult (climbing ropes, handstands etc)
- Venting frustration and relieving stress
- Great at shedding weight
- Testing yourself against previous versions of you
- Great friends to share the journey with, from all walks of life
- Great instructors to show you the path
- Motivation to see it through
- Ability to defend yourself
- Massive confidence increase

This book wouldn't exist without my martial arts career which is why I can't sell you on it enough. I implore you to find your physical outlet. It doesn't matter what it is as long as it motivates you.

If you live in, or are visiting Australia contact me with the details at the back of this book. I'm more than happy to introduce you at the gym.

Next Steps

So far I have discussed nutrition, exercise and provided a guideline for the first couple of months. Now we need to continue the good work and establish a framework to return to when the going gets tough.

Step 2 Energy Budget

After the initial 8 weeks it is time to control your energy intake with the informed choices gained from the above nutritional info. This is where you have a daily energy allowance, and stick to it. This doesn't work if you justify to yourself why you went over the budget today. It will too easily slip into a habit of eating more than you are allocated. It does take some discipline and willpower, covered in later chapters.

For the first month you are experimenting with your daily budget. From www.8700.com.au or similar sites you will have obtained your energy range. Start somewhere in the middle of the two values. Stick with that value for one week, see how you feel and measure your weight. If you are feeling low energy and weak then increase the allowance by 200kj for the next week. If you put on weight then drop it by 500kj. It should take about a month to figure out the best value for you.

Stick with this stable value for a month. Doing so should drop a fair amount of weight off you. This is great but does mean you have to adjust your daily budget again. Every month recalculate your budget according to your new weight. It should drop by 50kj to 500kj.

It's important to not go too fast. Starving yourself will not speed up weight loss but will hamper it as your body will hold onto fat cells, not knowing when fuel will be replenished. You have spent your entire life building to this point. It won't be reversed in a few weeks. As with anything worth doing, it's worth taking your time to do it right from the start.

Get yourself a notepad, mobile phone app or spreadsheet on your computer to track your energy consumption. I've included a sample at the back of the book. It doesn't take long to get into the habit of tracking protein, fat, carbs, fibre, sugars and sodium however it is less critical to do that for the first two months. The more data we can collect however, the easier the next steps will be. This data tracking will be maintained until you complete Step 5 Moderation for the first time.

Treat this process as research into your health. You are running observational experiments with your food intake. That appealed to me due to my scientific curiosity. If that doesn't appeal to you tie it to anything that motivates you. If sport tracking is your love, then create a spreadsheet with labels that match with sports stats. Energy budget is the opponent's score. You win by getting the closest to it without going over. There are multitudes of ways to see this data so it isn't boring to collate. Find a method that suits your interests to make it enjoyable and you'll get the most out of it.

Also step up your exercise once you have the stable energy value. Towards the end of the book I'll share some great exercise routines that build intensity as you get lighter and stronger. They don't fall directly in line with the meal steps as it depends on your individual progress and conditioning.

Step 3 Review Habits

Now is the time to really focus on our eating habits. The simplest way to do this is also quite confronting. Write down everything you are eating and drinking by name and the time you consume it. Remember to include everything such as cooking oils, condiments and spices. You'll be amazed at how much these additions impact your energy and nutrient budget.

It also helps to note down any particular thoughts or feelings you have at that moment as well. This is in conjunction with Step 2 Energy Budget, and should overlap it no more than 6 months after you begin that. You'll only need to do this additional tracking for a week or two so I suggest doing it as soon as you have your stable energy value and stuck to it for a month. This means roughly four months after you have started the journey.

This serves several purposes:

First, it highlights everything you are consuming and helps find groups you can eliminate one at a time. For me the biggest two groups were soft-drinks especially Coke, and lollies. Seeing these puts your habits into perspective and will likely make you feel upset or quite down on yourself. This is natural but a great and important step in the path. Feeling bad about where you are is a motivator to ensure you don't remain there for the rest of your life.

Second, noting the times down you can see at what point of the day you are more susceptible to snacking or overeating. We can then tackle these influences one at a time and try to see why we are eating more at those points. This may require a friend, life coach or psychologist to help identify and remedy the issues. Knowing they are present is a great first step in correcting them.

Third, understanding our emotional journey is key to realising why we are overeating. If you grab a chocolate bar every time you feel frustrated then we have a target to aim at. We can then focus on altering your response to frustration so it doesn't involve food. This is also where a life coach can greatly assist, as it can be difficult to figure it out on your own.

A book can't cover all the variables but I'll include a few in later chapters. I have contact details at the end of this book if you want to utilise my services in this area.

This is also a great time to dive into the charisma section presented later in this book. The negativity you may feel from having your food habits highlighted can be offset by improving interactions with others. Having charisma goals along with eating and exercise ones will help push you through plateaus as well.

The final point of this step is to add a 5 minute session at the start of each day to write down what you are grateful for. At the end of the day think about all the good things that happened to you, no matter how small. Then talk about these good points with your partner, friends or family when they ask how your day was. If we only focus on the negative it is very hard to turn things around in a positive light.

Step 4 The Elimination Round

Armed with the knowledge from Step 3 Review Habits, the next step is to remove one group of food or drink at a time. While maintaining the good habits we are establishing from the 8-week guide and sticking to our energy budget, for the next month remove the entire chosen group completely.

In my case I removed not only Coke but all caffeine from my diet. On top of Coke I also had energy drinks daily. I don't drink tea or coffee but assuming you do then these have to go as well. Replace them with water or coconut water. There are herbal teas without caffeine that might suit your palate as well.

The easiest way to do this is to have your chosen replacement always on hand. Get a 1 to 2 litre water bottle and fill it at the start of the day. Having it on your work desk and within easy reach is critical. Anytime you feel the need to drink caffeine, take a long swig of water and wait 5 minutes. The urge will usually pass.

The craving for caffeine or sugar will cause headaches for the first few days to a week. This is normal and you may feel grumpy. This is where your chosen activity helps. When you have a headache focus on whatever training you will be doing that day. With a little willpower you can ignore the headaches easily. See later in this book for willpower strategies.

In the case of caffeine you will see benefits of removing it in a little over a week. Your sleep patterns will be far better. You won't wake up tired and you'll have more energy. You may also have lost a bit of weight from a significant drop in sugar intake, assuming you have Coke or add sugar to coffee.

Add in the challenge that each week you must try a new healthier beverage you have never had before. I chose vegetable juice, different fruit juice (freshly squeezed) and even some kava from Fiji. For many of you coconut water will be a new experience. This is basically a natural energy drink without the stimulants and sugars added to manufactured ones. These new drinks offer a mental distraction from the one you have cut out, and help as replacements when cravings kick in.

At the end of the month, challenge yourself to remain free of the chosen group for as long as possible. You are now able to add the removed items back in, but in moderation. For example you can have two cans of Coke a week maximum. However to help with future goals make this an irregular pattern. Keep the re-introduction minimal as it will speed up your weight loss and strengthen your willpower. You don't want to get all the benefits of a caffeine free life and then hook yourself back onto it. One or two cans a week will give you the taste you enjoy but shouldn't impact your diet or sleep. Just don't have them on the same day, at night or as a means to wake up. Lunchtime is a good option. You could also switch to the zero sugar option, saving a massive hit on your energy budget.

Adding it back in helps maintain your willpower however really notice how you feel after consuming the removed item. You'll likely find you don't really enjoy it like you used to. It may take a few times of removing and adding back in to kick the habit completely. The second you realise you are falling back into old patterns, tell yourself you deserve better and remove the item immediately. A life coach will help kick it to the curb for good.

Repeat this every month for three months, each time removing a new group. Take the opportunity to replace the removed group with something healthy you have never tried before.

When adding items back in look for a better choice instead of reverting back to old habits. For example, instead of eating milk chocolate, try dark chocolate or even better raw chocolate. Raw chocolate doesn't have added dairy and is naturally gluten free for those with celiac disease.

We are training ourselves to try new things in place of the poor choices we have made up to this point. You should find something healthier that you like and then use it as a substitute. Remember the ultimate goal is to reach our target weight and enjoy life. I don't want to count kilojoules for the rest of my life. I want to enjoy cake and chocolate from time to time. But I needed to establish healthy baseline habits and have a safety net so I don't return to the old poor choices.

For the longest time I knew I hated broccoli. I knew this from the moment I saw it as a 6 year old. I never actually ate any, but simply from the look and smell I decided I hated it. I can rattle off a list of foods that fall into this category that will fill a notepad. However as an adult I challenged myself to try new things to distract me from the craving of junk food. What I discovered is that these foods actually tasted fine. Plus they filled me far more than the crap I had been eating. This works best when sugar is removed as your taste alters dramatically. With constant sugar, foods that don't contain it seem bland. Removing sugar from the equation allows the full taste experience to shine through.

Gaining this understanding first hand is vital as we begin to experience a healthy lifestyle and alter our mentality.

Step 5 Moderation

After three months of subtraction, take a month to restore balance. This is where we continue with the good habits but piece by piece add the junk snacks in a limited manner. We have to train ourselves to still enjoy our indulgences but not let them take over.

In this stage, limit your subtracted substances to two a week for snacks and drinks, and once a fortnight for takeout. It won't be the end of the world if you break this limit by a little, but try to figure out why you did similar to Step 3 Review Habits.

Take note of how your body, weight and energy levels react after eating the poor food choice. You should feel off, weighed down or tired when eating too much junk food. While eating a pizza may feel like heaven at the time, later that day or by the next you will feel drained. Your stomach will feel crappy and you'll likely need a bowel movement to begin feeling better.

This step is important to gain insight into healthy eating that we couldn't do until now. With the poor food choices removed, our body functions with efficiency. It quickly gets used to untainted fuel and craves more. If you add in the junk again it's like you've put ethanol into your unleaded car. You can still function but not at the same level as the correct fuel. Once we can recognise how food alters our body feel, we are prepared to add in the high octane fuel to truly soar.

This stage is a great place to be as we can really feel how our food choices impact our health. You will remain here the longest as the weight drops off. Anytime you reach a plateau, alternate between Steps 4 and 5 for a few weeks at a time.

Once you have reached a stable process between Steps 4 and 5, you can stop counting your energy consumption. You should have ample experience to understand what you should be eating and can identify the best options.

Congratulations on achieving this much. You have come a long way and deserve applause. There is however one more step to go and it's a doozy.

Depending on your starting weight, activity levels, motivations and number of plateaus this equilibrium

Overweight to Fighting Weight

could last anywhere from 8 months to 5 years before you are ready to move onto Step 6 The Ultimate Push.

<u>Step 6 The Ultimate Push</u>

I'm not going to blow smoke up your butt, step 6 will suck. It will take you far beyond your comfort zone and you will want to track me down and break my face in.

However it is necessary if you want to reach the pinnacle of what you can achieve. If you are happy continuing with steps 4 and 5 for the rest of your life and the levels it brings you to, then fine. We don't all need to be top level athletes or swimsuit models.

I do however recommend you try this at least once. Shaking up your comfortable status can improve motivation. As the saying goes, familiarity breeds contempt. The more familiar and comfortable you are with your weight loss, the easier it is to get bored and revert to old habits.

The Ultimate Push will test everything you've learnt; it will try to break you mentally. Don't let it. Gaining the ability to persevere through this step will create a far stronger version of you, both physically and mentally. You can use this to achieve anything you want in life as you'll understand how to fight through adversity.

You will need to understand the goal setting, motivation and willpower sections coming up to get you through this step, however I am including it now to show you what the end point looks like.

This is also important as the final 10kgs can be the toughest to lose. You could continue for a year and slowly burn it off while draining your motivation; or you could work your arse off for a month and see amazing results now.

If you have any medical issues please take this book to your trusted medical practitioners and show them what you are intending to do. You may need some alterations based on your specific circumstances. I have done this myself so am not asking you to do anything I wouldn't do. The knowledge comes from professional athletes and sports trainers which I have modified for my own needs. It does work when you give it your best.

Do not perform Step 6 more than twice per year, and even then make sure it is at least 6 months after your previous session. Once complete go back to Steps 4 and 5. The idea of The Ultimate Push is to do this once near the end of your journey to get rid of the stubborn fat remnants, and then maintain that new weight. Done right you shouldn't need to do this more than once.

With that doom and gloom out of the way, let's begin.

The Rules

This restrictive food plan will last for 30 days. You will be having three meals a day plus two snacks. You are only allowed water but can drink as much of it as you like. Items not listed below are not allowed for this 30 day period.

For each meal you will pick a source of protein and pair it with a source of carbs from the lists below. Serving sizes are critical here. For protein it should be the size of your hand, without fingers. For carbs it will be two cups for vegies, three cups for leafy greens (spinach, lettuce etc), one piece of fruit, or a handful for small fruit like grapes. Nuts are to be no more than one handful per day.

Protein Sources

Beef, chicken, duck, fish, eggs, lamb, seafood, turkey, protein powder, quinoa, tofu, beans (pinto or kidney).

Cooking oil you can use is avocado oil, coconut oil, flax oil or olive oil.

Carbohydrate Sources

Vegetables:

Asparagus, bok choy, broccoli, Brussel sprouts, cabbage, cauliflower, cucumber, eggplant, kale, kai-lan, lettuce, mushrooms, onions, peppers, spinach, Swiss chard, tomato, zucchini.

Fruit:

Apple, apricot, banana, berries, cantaloupe, cherries, coconut, grapefruit, grapes, guava, kiwi fruit, lemon, lime, mango, melon, orange, papaya, peach, pear, pineapple, plum.

Nuts (snacks):

Almonds, brazil nuts, cashews, flax seeds, chia seeds, macadamia nuts, peanuts, pecans, pine nuts, pistachios, pumpkin seeds, sesame seeds, sunflower seeds, walnuts.

All nuts are to be raw. This means unroasted, unsalted and not baked as these processes generally add unwanted ingredients.

Meals

Breakfast and lunch will consist of protein, fruit and vegetables from the options above. Dinner is protein and vegetables only. Between each main meal you will have your snack, and water is had through the entire day.

Overweight to Fighting Weight

I'd recommend taking a daily multi-vitamin supplement to ensure you are getting all your required micro-nutrients. Again seek advice from your trusted medical professionals for any specific concerns.

Cardio

You will also need to exercise two or three times per week at high intensity, never on consecutive days.

An exercise bike with a heart rate monitor is great here. You will want your heart rate to be over 160BPM, and to take the bike to a pace of 90RPM or higher. This should last for 30 minutes to an hour. Ensure you eat a meal after this exercise, within 10 to 20 minutes of completing it.

Before breakfast, if possible, is the recommended time. Any exercise that gets your heart rate over 160BMP will suffice as long as it can be sustained for at least 30 minutes. Please consult your doctor before starting these exercises to ensure your personal condition can handle it. Assuming you have followed the exercise guide below you should be capable of this.

Precautions

As you will be energy depleted for this month, it will be best to have an energy gel on hand when exercising. Energy gels provide a hit of carbs that are designed to enter your system rapidly. They may be required to get you through the workout.

Don't have more than one per session however and ensure your heart rate is already up (you are sweating from exertion) before taking it otherwise your energy will crash. Energy gels can be found at the supermarket, at cycling stores and most gyms.

Always take account of how you are feeling during these sessions. If you are tired you can push through, but if you are dizzy or seeing spots it is time to stop, hydrate and eat.

Results

With the food restrictions and exercise above, you should lose between 5kg and 15kg in these 30 days as long as you stick with it. There are no cheat days here. Once this is done congratulate yourself for all your hard work. Actually take time to celebrate: buy that coat you were wanting; go to a movie you've been holding out for; invite friends over for a gaming session. It doesn't matter what it is as long as you acknowledge how far you have come. Just don't ruin your progress by celebrating with pizza and ice-cream.

Having experienced this once, you will never want to go through it again. That itself should motivate you to maintain your reduced weight.

The first time I did this was one of the hardest things I did, but it taught me a lot about myself. It made me realise the human body doesn't need anywhere near as much food as we generally provide it. The biggest hurdle to get over was the understanding I would be constantly hungry. This state made me agitated and quick to temper.

Funnily enough that only lasted about 10 days. My body got used to the depleted fuel and altered how it was treated. My exercise and martial arts training were hard for the first couple of weeks but with the energy gels and determination I pushed through.

By the final week I was used to the lower energy and was beginning to treat it as normal. I wouldn't have been able to compete effectively but could get through the training without issue.

Overweight to Fighting Weight

Once the food was allowed back in as per step 5, I could feel the extra energy surging, impatient to be utilised. That feeling lasted about a month, which gave me time to still enjoy it when the competition finally arrived.

To get through Step 6 The Ultimate Push you'll need the focus that goals, motivation and willpower can provide. Read on for insight into those.

<u>Understanding Motivation</u>

Staying motivated in any extended activity can be a challenge. In sport it's critical to have coaches and guides with great technical knowledge, as well as the ability to inspire and push you towards your full potential. Losing weight isn't much different, though it can be harder to find a great coach.

This doesn't only refer to sport, but to life. How many times have you tried something but failed to remain motivated? Maybe you quit because it was too hard, frustrating or you had too much pressure to succeed? Keeping motivation is difficult when we can no longer see a reason to enjoy an activity. Perhaps your success has pushed you into a higher level of competition and the intensity is no longer fun.

Remember you are your own competition. Shedding 15kg in two months feels great, but you can feel angry at yourself for only dropping 8kg in the next three months. This is fine however; you are still removing the weight and getting closer to your goals. Weight loss isn't a constant line.

I have experienced many a dint in motivation in my life but nothing comes to mind more than when I played competitive pool (8-ball). In this comp there were 10 divisions, with div 1 being the highest. I started in div 8 with an average team. I had a few friends in divisions 2 and 3 and filled in for them on occasion due to illness or work. My skill set was thus significantly higher than where I was playing but I had little pressure so could enjoy it more. I switched teams and divisions a few times as player's commitments and priorities changed. I remained in division 5 for several years and we all generally had fun with challenging opponents. That changed when we won the grand final and were thus forced into div 4.

It started out OK, but our new opponents took everything too seriously. The pressure to play your best was enormous. If you had one or two poor shots you quickly lost. The enjoyment plummeted not only for me but for the entire team. We disbanded after a single season at div 4 rather than taint our enjoyment of the game. This is something everyone needs to address at some point. Our reason for playing was for a fun night out with friends and some good competition. As soon as that changed our motivation sagged. Recognising this we made an informed choice and now still enjoy a good social game.

I have struggled with motivation for losing weight; there have been times I just couldn't be bothered training or going to work. I was grumpy and just wanted some chocolate or a cheesecake. But thinking about why you are doing something can restore motivation during difficult times, and keep you from disappointment in yourself.

To succeed and cope with the demands of that success you must enjoy what you are doing, remember where you started and maintain perspective. Obviously if we aren't enjoying that activity (sports) or the results (less weight, bigger muscles etc) then we can't see why we should continue. Take a look back on just how far you have come from when it all started.

Don't focus on the fact you gained 4kg over Christmas, remember that you lost 20kg this year. Also know where you are and what you are trying to achieve. Don't worry about the struggles at the end point when you are only half way. Your plans and goals should have an understanding of the end result but concentrate on the obstacle in front of you now.

Maintain control of your life. Figure out your priorities for how you spend your time. Take care of your needs, and that of your loved ones, first. You should have time for rest and relaxation, proper nutrition, life's simple pleasures, physical activities and anything else you consider important. It's your life and your time so spend it wisely to make the best of it.

Create a plan on how to deal with demands. Life can't be planned in detail and the unexpected will crop up. Expect that this will happen and make a systematic plan on dealing with it. Figure out how many different demands you can reasonably tackle at various points in the year and don't take on more. School holidays may see you cutting back on the gym to take care of the kids. Establish a black out on your time when you are not available for external demands. Advise those important to you and stick to it. Demands and priorities change, accept what is important to you and let others slip by.

Remember what you did to get to this point. The process and activities you stuck to in order to get where you are now clearly worked. Don't throw them away due to a few bad weeks. Remember the basics and reflect on what allowed you to succeed. Working hard, taking adequate rest, enjoyment of the activities, belief in yourself and your coaches, mental and physical preparedness and accepting new challenges are all required to stay positive and get the results you expect.

Figure out how to avoid distractions. Set your focus on what you can control and what you want to achieve. If you can't control something there is no point worrying about it. Plan on how you can work around these uncontrollable issues but don't let them distract you. Draw on the expertise of others when planning. Other people have faced similar issues as you, and your coach has overcome greater obstacles. Lean on their friendship and wisdom. If you can't find someone hit me up via the contact details at the back of the book.

If you are really struggling with emotional and mental wellbeing you can utilise a Life Coach for managing thoughts and feelings, and work with you to discover methods to cope with your life's many challenges. Focus on what is important and you'll make it through.

Motivation Triggers

Motivational changes are normal and occur for everyone at some point. High level athletes and fitness gurus are not immune and have had many lulls over their career. I took a decade to get the results I wanted and I guarantee my motivation waned more times than I can count. One aspect of their success and my own is that we understand our own motivations and can identify when it changes.

If you can understand what triggers a change in motivation you have more control over how to handle it and remain motivated when things get tough. To begin it is best to figure out what it feels like to be highly motivated.

High Motivation

Think about your behaviour and how you feel when you are highly motivated and performing at your best. Grab a piece of paper or open a text editor on your computer and pick a situation you experienced high motivation. Visualise the specific moment; step into your own body, see what you saw, hear what you heard and feel what you felt. Write down everything you notice, describe your attitude and actions, jot down any thoughts or feelings you recall having at that time. A qualified Life Coach can anchor this awesome feeling so you can trigger it whenever you need.

This process establishes a target baseline of where you want to be. You have already been at this highly motivated peak so emulating that in the future can get you out of your funk.

For me this was at the 2013 Australian BJJ Championships. I travelled to Sydney and at the time my coach was unavailable to join me. I was the only representative of my gym but thankfully my wife was with me. I entered in my weight division and the open weight division as I wasn't going all that way to come back empty handed.

I remember thinking I wouldn't let down my coach by not performing at my best. The morning of the event I was calm and joking around with my wife. The hotel was a 20 minute walk from the venue and from the moment I saw other people walking around with gym bags my brain switched into combat mode. I didn't speak and had laser focus. I visualised my fights from the point of walking on the mat, going over taking my opponents to the ground and submitting them in a variety of methods. I saw their counters to my moves and saw how I could capitalise on that. In short I dissected the fight and its multiple avenues before even seeing the venue.

During the fights themselves there were several times my opponents gained the upper hand, but I didn't think negatively. I knew I could escape the situation and turned their initial minor victories into crushing defeats. One of my opponents was up on points by a large margin until I quickly escaped a tight submission, countered while he scrambled to retain hold and choked him out for the win. He angrily smacked the ground and acted like a two year old that was denied an ice-cream. That served to fuel my calm as even if I lost the next match I refused to behave like an ungrateful infant. Dealing with defeat is hard but you still need to face yourself in the mirror.

Being at a motivational high ensured my techniques were razor sharp, that I could clinically setup my opponents and I could react quicker. My dual gold medals at the event were in no small part due to the high motivation I had to win. Now that I have that understanding, I can aim to duplicate that in the future whenever I'm low.

Low Motivation

Everyone experiences lows and it greatly affects performance. There are many factors for low motivation including injury, anxiety, stress from work, personal conflicts, a slump in performance, other people outperforming you and vastly more.

At low motivation something in the situation needs to change. The Martial Arts have taught me a lot, but a key aspect is that moving an obstacle such as a strong opponent's arm is prohibitively exhausting. But moving yourself into a different angle of attack can expose a weakness. Imagine two people pushing against each other with all their might. There is no movement in either direction as the opposite forces are mostly equal. You can't make any headway, but if you stop pushing back and pivot to the side their inertia propels them into the area you vacated. Their power is focussed forward but you are now attacking from the side.

At times of low motivation you need to pivot to the side and tackle the problem from a different angle.

Identifying when your motivation is waning before you hit the bottom is important. Escaping a submission at its most effective point is damn hard. Recognising when you are in danger of being submitted and countering before you are in trouble is the key to staying in the game. You may not win from escaping but you definitely won't lose. Staying in the game means you still have a shot at victory, and I've won many competitions against dominant opponents by simply staying in the game until I could find a chink in their armour.

An equivalent in weight loss is recognising when you crave junk food. If you know frustration propels you towards chocolate, then work to pinpoint what makes you frustrated and attack it before it becomes a problem.

Understanding yourself during periods of low motivation helps you make effective decisions and move toward positive activities to enhance that situation. After you have a negative thought or action think of better ways you can handle it in the future.

Read over these examples of some low motivation thoughts and mark down all that you have experienced:

- I'm not sure I can do that
- I'm too injured
- I'm too fat
- I have no energy
- I'm bored
- Why wasn't I selected for the team? I must be useless
- My coach is pushing me too hard
- My partners are improving far quicker than me
- My time training is interfering with my relationship and friends
- I'm so hungry
- Work is really hectic right now and I can't focus on other things

Overweight to Fighting Weight

- I'm doing everything wrong
- I'm not getting enough attention from the coach
- I'm not good at this
- This is too hard
- One chocolate bar won't hurt
- This is taking too long
- I should quit
- I'm not having any fun
- Why am I bothering?
- Is this the right thing for me at this point in my life?

As soon as you have a thought similar to the above you should realise this is a red flag towards lowering your motivation. At this point you need to pivot to the side and return to focus. That is easier said than done so let's take this personal analysis further.

What am I thinking?

Motivation is all in your head. The body will move when the mind tells it to. You can push through obstacles with determination when your body is weak. So figuring out how and what you think are critical to identifying highs and lows and how to address any problems.

Same as with high times, low points have many factors that can be brought back to thoughts, emotions and behaviours.

I've thought some very negative things during training sessions. I've though it's boring as I have done the repetitions a thousand times. I've bummed myself out knowing I'm overweight or unfit. I've been tired and wanted to find an excuse to stop the training session, even if it meant faking an injury.

If I let each of these negative thoughts affect me I wouldn't train at all. In every case I found a way to push through in part due to my stubborn nature. I'm not saying I'm immune to low motivation, I've spent months in a funk and struggled to extract myself. But stray thoughts like these should trigger a response and are an opportunity to self-evaluate. Has something altered in your life adding pressure? Are you physically exhausted and need a break for a few days? Has your diet changed, or could it change? Are you stepping up your training and haven't taken all factors into account for time, effort and energy requirements? Do you need to revisit your daily energy budget?

Your coaches, senior students, friends and family can help with many of these. I guarantee they have had very similar issues and can help. Find a friend that has achieved some sort of success, even if it isn't in weight loss. Talk to them about your issues and I guarantee they have had a similar experience. Just talking about it can bring perspective.

This is one reason why it's great to do tasks such as losing weight with a group of people. Each of you can motivate the others as a team. Your life partner is a great place to start. It's another reason I recommend doing a sport or self-defence. You have access to a wide variety of people you wouldn't normally connect with, and they all share issues with motivation. Utilise them and help others when needed.

I feel...

What we think will influence how we feel. If we think negatively then the feelings will follow suit. This is why we need to realise what we think and change it before it affects us further. Often when I have these negative thoughts I immediately shout in my mind "I deserve better than this" and rework the thought. This stops it impacting my feelings in any substantial way.

For example if I've put on 3kg I might think I'm fat and I can't do this anymore. I would then shout the above mantra to myself and change the thought to "I'm going to alter my meals for tomorrow." This way I didn't give the depressed feeling a chance to settle and I made an action plan for fixing the situation. I may fail in the execution or I may succeed but as long as I identify the red flags and do something to halt negativity in its tracks, I can refocus.

Another great method is to simply acknowledge the thought, thank it for bringing the low motivational state to your attention, then tell it to sod off or shut up. Follow this up immediately with a positively focussed statement that counters the unhelpful thought.

I've found there is a small delay between having a thought and experiencing a related emotion. By immediately denying the thought and changing it to something positive you can stave off feelings that will alter your actions. This needs to occur as close to the point of the negative thought as possible, otherwise the feelings kick in and cause additional negativity. Don't allow yourself to be spiralled into the depths of the poorly motivated just because a single stray thought snowballed.

The below are some examples of feelings that can greatly impact motivation. If you are experiencing any of them try to figure out its source and address the issue. The feeling was likely seeded by a stray thought and took root to weaken your wall of motivation.

- Anxious
- Ashamed
- Confused
- Discouraged
- Embarrassed
- Frustrated
- Guilty
- Helpless
- Irritated
- Lonely
- Nervous
- Sad
- Scared
- Stressed
- Weary

Having these feelings is normal and nothing to be ashamed of, but by understanding they are triggers you can get control of your mental state and achieve great things.

Behave yourself

How you think and feel in a given situation influences how you react and behave. This may cause changes that are helpful or a hindrance. Obviously you want to do whatever is helpful and avoid self-sabotage.

I've mentioned that thoughts lead to feelings, which alter actions. The inverse is true as well, so changing your behaviour can tackle your negative thoughts and emotions from a different angle.

There are times I've felt like crap, thought everything was failing in martial arts, I didn't feel I was progressing and I had put on a few kilos. I even told my coach I wanted to scrap my entire game plan and start again from scratch. I wasn't in the frame of mind to alter my thoughts and feelings. Instead I changed my actions. I switched to training at a different time of day. I scheduled a private lesson with my coach. I dived into coaching others and changed my standard meals to gain some variety. Within a short time I got back on track, dropped several kilos and improved performance. My motivation was restored and I kept going for almost a year before the next slump approached.

Overweight to Fighting Weight

The following shows a short selection of negative and positive behaviours that you may have done or witnessed in others. Recognising your behaviour as negative is the first step to making positive change.

Negative Behaviours	Positive Behaviours
Minimal effort and intensity at training	Fully engaged and high training effort
Skipped weights leg day	Hunted for more challenging tasks
Left training early to avoid speaking with the coach	Was candid with coach about my problem areas and discussed extensively
Angry at self for failing to understand a technique	Aided others when the coach was occupied elsewhere
Consumed chocolate when feeling down	Didn't buy any junk food with the weekly groceries
Felt bored so ate a few snacks	Felt bored so weeded the garden

Now that we can identify our behaviour we can work on ensuring it's as positive as possible. I have often experienced negative thoughts, feelings and behaviour during training. Mostly I have been able to get around them by focusing on my goals. I also have the benefit of world champion fighters and an Olympic wrestler as coaches. I don't want them to think I'm wasting their time and effort training me, so push through my negativity to avoid their disappointment.

Those that know me well understand meeting new people has been a challenge for me, and I have struggled to remain comfortable in social interactions especially where there are a lot of strangers. Small talk seems pointless and I quickly slipped into silence.

When I speak to people I speak with a purpose so cut through all the unnecessary chit chat. That made me seem abrupt. The reason I'm telling you is because I identified this as normal behaviour for me. I now make an effort by noticing when I behave in this way and go out of my way to make at least minimal small talk before I get down to business. For me this was challenging. Sincerity is difficult to fake so I have to actually be sincere in asking how your day was and be interested in your answer.

The thing I have found with doing this is it's easier each time. I began thinking about how I influence others and what I can do as a team member. I ask my coach how I can help others and how I can improve advising during and after a fight. I'm not only focussed on my own training but want to see my team mates succeed.

Identifying my undesired behaviour and seeking change influenced how I think and feel and now I am a better instructor and coach because of it. I have digested hundreds of hours of information on changing mindsets, improving charisma, meeting people, coaching and many other self-improvement topics. All of this came from identifying negative behaviour and doing something positive to change it. None of it would have been possible if I didn't force myself down the road of massive weight loss.

Factors affecting motivation

Clearly understanding typical situations, thoughts, feelings and behaviours when your motivation is low, allows you to enhance your future motivation. Work to alter at least one aspect so you can influence the others. Again we can pivot to the side and tackle the problem from a different angle. The main changes we can make are generally: to your environment; to your thoughts about the situation; or to your behaviour.

Making one of these alterations when your motivation is low will aid in taking control over yourself and enhance your motivation. This is a powerful factor of success at any endeavour. Mastering this will mean you can achieve anything you set your sights on.

Key Advice

Stop thinking about bad performance or not having enough energy. Remember you are measuring against your previous self. Coaches and weight loss buddies are here to help you achieve your goals, not berating you for failing. We all lose motivation at times, and we all have poor performance days. As long as you keep striving to do better, you will.

You will often feel like you are under performing and set a lot of pressure on yourself to improve. You aren't performing as poorly as you feel. We are our own worst critic. Remove your feelings of guilt for underperforming. Not all training sessions can be at your maximum output. Not all weeks can be weight loss records. We need time to recover, time to reflect and re-align goals.

If you are frustrated by performing a technique in a suboptimal way, just go with it and try again. That is why we rep. You don't need it perfect every time, but we do continually strive to improve from the last few reps. If you get one or two wrong, you will fix it on the next. Don't behave as if it's the end of the world.

Focussing on the negative will waste your time as you vent anger and frustration. Instead simply accept it wasn't the best version and improve upon it in the next rep. To align this with weight loss, each meal is a new rep. Each day or week is a new set of reps. Accept the past and strive for doing better next time.

To paraphrase my coach John, we should be unrelenting in our unattainable pursuit of perfection. It is impossible to achieve pure perfection but that doesn't mean we can't skim the edge of it.

Summary

Periods of low motivation are normal for everyone throughout their life. Learn to recognise these periods and their corresponding thoughts, feelings and behaviours as this helps to effectively manage motivation when the going gets tough. Those that can recognise low periods and take positive action have the most success.

Remind yourself to achieve success rather than simply avoid failure. Think about your focus. Which of the following areas of focus will make you happier?

1. What you can control
2. What you can't control

1. What you have in life
2. What you don't have in life

1. The future
2. The present
3. The past

In all groups of focus, number 1 will make you happier and help keep you motivated. In the last group you should also focus on the present so you can turn it into the future you desire.

Overweight to Fighting Weight

Thoughts, feelings and behaviours influence each other. If they are all negative, change one of them to improve the rest.

Change the angle of attack to get a different grasp of the issue. Conditions don't determine your destiny, decisions do.

Examine old thinking habits and open yourself to new experiences and challenges. You will be surprised at how far you can reach.

<u>Goal Setting</u>

There is no magic bullet for goal setting. No one method can cater to every person, every situation or every end result. The following is one method that has worked well for me in a lot of areas. The main objective of setting goals is to give our desires life. Having them written down or stated in a formal manner can be enough to surge us forward. Many of us need that extra push however and the methods below aim to provide that.

Setting attainable goals is crucial in sports, weight loss and for most major projects in your life. The process doesn't need to be onerous but it does need sufficient thought to understand what we need to do to accomplish the goals.

Setting a goal is more of a process cycle. The steps flow into each other but never stop. The process restarts with your new status as the starting point for further improvement. The basic steps are:

- Decide what you want to achieve
- Plan how you will get to that point
- Work towards the goal
- Monitor and evaluate

There are three main parts to your goal: the grand vision; short term goals and action goals. Each are important to understand your path to success.

Grand Vision Goals

To start with we define the vision, or more simply the end state that we want to achieve. This may be to reach a specific weight, to be selected for the national team in your sport or to publish your first novel. At this stage you don't need to know how to get there, just that it's your desire to reach it.

We want to keep all of these goals as positive as possible. Stating I want to lose 30kgs is a great goal however it is stated negatively. Assuming you are 120kg at present, a more positive version is to state I want to reach 90kgs. It is a small adjustment but can greatly impact your motivation. Knowing what you are aiming for, and keeping it in mind in a positive light, helps the climb out of low motivation.

Keep these goals to a smaller timeframe. Planning ahead more than a few years will make working towards it that much harder. As it is so far in the future it can be difficult to see each milestone along the way. We can always adjust these down the line.

Stepping Stone Goals

These are the main steps you need in order to reach your Grand Vision Goals. They include a specific area to improve and a time frame in which to reach it.

Break these down into 90 day chunks. What can you do in the next 90 days to get a decent step closer to your grand vision? Doing it in 90 day segments allows you to focus on one aspect with a short period of time. We build momentum by knocking off smaller tasks and getting a pile of them. Looking back on our achievements helps break through plateaus and low motivation. Three months is ample time to see real changes and realistically plan our actions over that span.

Continuing with the examples above, stepping stone goals to achieve in the next 90 days could be to reach a specific weight (eg 112kg), stop opponents from easily passing my Guard, or finish writing five chapters.

Armed with these we can figure out how to build towards them each day.

Action Goals

This is the most important, as action goals tell you how you will achieve your Stepping Stone Goals. These goals represent the specific actions you need to do today or this week to reach your Stepping Stone Goals and eventually your Grand Vision Goals. When setting Action Goals ensure they are positively framed and SMART, Specific, Measurable, Action based, Realistic and Time limited

Being specific helps focus on the tasks you need to do to achieve your goals. You need something to measure them by to tell if you have achieved it. They need to highlight the action or behaviour you require. They have to be challenging but realistic to achieve otherwise missing the high demand will increase frustration and generally cause failure. Finally you need to set a time limit on the task to stay motivated and provide a date for progress review.

While I like the SMART system, there are limitations to it. People can get stuck with ensuring a realistic target for example, and not set a goal to truly push themselves. In shedding the kilos, dropping 10kg in a week is unrealistic and a potential health risk. Dropping 1kg in a week might be too easy and can bring cheating with chocolate as you have already reached the goal. Dropping 3kg in a week will be difficult but in the realm of possibility, especially at the early stages.

Always strive to have your goals set out of easy reach, but not so far that you have to break something to get there.

Overweight to Fighting Weight

This isn't the only aspect needed however. We also need to build a few success levels for the goal.

Good, Better, Best

We want a good, better and best target to aim for. A Good target may be to write 800 words today. A Better target is 1500 words and the Best target is over 2000 words.

Each one will bring you closer to your goal but the Best is clearly the winner in getting stuff done. If you only achieve the Good goal today you have still achieved something. Now you can strive to better it tomorrow.

You should strive to achieve one Good (minor), one Better (medium) and One Best (major) goal every day. Aim for finishing the Best goal first, that way you have a great start to the day and can look back on a significant achievement. You should limit the amount of areas your goals focus on. Over three months you can work on maybe three different Stepping Stone Goals. More than that will take too much focus away from your day.

When we change focus it takes our brain time to adjust to the new task, the more we switch in a day the more time required to get back into the flow. Three 90 day projects at once is the sweet spot. It keeps you busy but it's not overwhelming. If you find three too challenging then drop it back to two or one. Just ensure the most important goal, the one that has the biggest impact and progress to your Grand Vision, is the one your work on first.

The key is to ask yourself two questions:
1) "What can I achieve in the next 90 days that brings me closer to my Grand Vision goal?"
2) "What can I do each day to ensure I get one step closer to that Stepping Stone 90 day goal?"

The answers will form the structure of your Action Goals.

Goals need to be malleable and continually evaluated. That mainly occurs in the Action Goals. The Grand Vision and Stepping Stone Goals rarely change once set.

If we struggle achieving a set result we may have to evaluate our targets. They may be too unrealistic to achieve at that point. Dropping them back a notch may be required for a few weeks until we can build up steam. To more easily do this, we think about our goal and make the measurable target the Better option. We can then raise and lower it to get the Best and Good goals respectively.

Some examples in regards to weight loss could be the following (15/20/30 would be Good of 15, Better of 20 and Best of 30).

- 15/20/30 minutes of high intensity (heart rate over 160bpm) exercise bike (over 85rpm) at least once every 3 days for this month.
- Consume soft drink can(s) 5/3/1 times per week for this month.
- Consume fast food 3/2/1 time(s) this month.
- Consume no more than 12/10/8% over my allotted energy budget for this week. Reduce that to 7/5/3% over for week 2, 4/0/-2% over for week 3 and 0/3/5% under for week 4. Evaluate new energy budget after week 4 then repeat.

Be as specific as possible. Narrow down the days and times you will do something if it's realistic to do so. Adding to the above you might specify you do the bike exercise on Monday, Wednesday and Friday at 7am. Or you will have a soft drink only on Saturday and Sunday at lunch.

Armed with this you have decided what you want, planned how to do it, can work towards it and measure your results. You will find your goals a lot easier to manage when breaking it down this way.

Don't put too much stress on yourself by having a large number of goals. You will burn out. These are 90 day sprints. If you can't fit something in this time around, add it in for the next 90 days. This keeps focus tight so you can really pin down a narrow area and get the most from it.

A good method to prevent committing to too much is every Sunday morning, brainstorm everything you could do in the week to get a step closer to your goals. Look for items that give the greatest benefit with the smallest amount of effort. Collect a handful of these and delay the rest for a week.

If the smaller impact items are time sensitive, but others can do them for you, think about hiring someone to help out. This will free up time to focus on what is critical to you, such as going to the gym. Fiverr.com is a great source for people willing to do work on the cheap. You get more quality the higher you pay but can get a lot of value. There are plenty of similar websites that offer the same services, but I've had a lot of success with Fiverr sellers.

Managing Willpower

Willpower is finite. It's the fuel in your tank, the mana bar in a video game. When it's depleted you can still function but not at peak efficiency. You will be sluggish and bad habits will sneak back in. Your mind has had enough and you will find ways to justify a little chocolate here, a soft drink there or fail to stop at just one slice of pizza.

It isn't just preventing poor behaviour that drains willpower. Spending time thinking about a decision before it is actually made is a massive drain to the tank.
Exerting your willpower is a big drain, like trying not to cry at a sad movie. Forcing feelings when you feel the opposite is draining as well, such as being out with friends and forcing yourself to feel happy when you are currently sad.

None of these things in themselves are a bad thing unless they form a habit; we just have to understand that they drain our Willpower Tank (WT). This prevents us being able to use it later when needed to stop eating crap. This is why we tend to break our goals or blow our food energy budget at night. The day has drained our WT and we need to recharge.

Food and sleep replenishes our WT, which is a double edged sword. We need willpower to not eat crap, but eating restores the same tank eating healthy depletes. We can strengthen our willpower and increase its capacity by using it, however it takes a long time to do so, especially when hungry, training, working and paying bills.

Mastery over your willpower does not mean you have an infinite tank. Mastery means using it efficiently and only when truly required, doing more with less. To help achieve this we can setup our life to drain willpower the least. Remember in the motivation section I mentioned we are happier to focus on things we can control. This helps build a structure based support system so we don't need to rely on our willpower.

To help me with this I have a standard breakfast, lunch and dinner menu. Breakfast is always a thick smoothie. I include a sachet of instant oats, a scoop of protein powder, water and frozen fruit. Blended up this creates a filling meal and I already have my serves of fruit out of the way. I also have not used any willpower before I start my workday as I have taken all thinking and decision making out of the equation.

Lunch is a wrap instead of bread, some meat such as chicken, leftover roast or slow cooked meat and some leafy greens. When I purchase the meat I always go with the cheapest option so I don't have to dwell on making a decision. I also like meals from providers such as YouFoodz. They create a lot of fresh, healthy options that you can toss in a microwave and enjoy in minutes. I always have a handful available and grab the topmost one for a meal that day.

Snacks are from a choice of four options which again I purchase based on the cheapest at the time of shopping. These are things like muesli bars, nuts, yoghurt and canned tuna.

Dinner is likewise a choice of a few different meals, and I make them based on whichever is closest to the top of the freezer. I generally include a type of meat, oven baked chips (no oil) and veggies such as corn or peas.

Throughout all of this I am not wasting time or my WT in deliberating about the choice. I don't need to make a decision because I put a system in place to do that for me. This system comes from the several things we can control to ensure willpower is there when required.

Build this system across all areas of your life that you can control. At work the first thing each day might be to fill your water bottle and answer your emails. At training you can create a warm up routine and stretching schedule to hit the ground running.

I have created a weekly schedule that I stick to consistently. Training times are set so when the time comes I know what I'm doing without thinking. I have times during the weekend where I only play games. Sunday morning is my main writing time. I don't need willpower to start these activities because it is simply what I do at that time.

The more we can take decisions and procrastination away, the more willpower we will have to use later.

Rapid Decisions

We need to work at making decisions quickly. Our brain doesn't care what the decision is, but the process involved in making it. Stop saying "I don't care" when asked to make a choice. When you say this your mind is still processing the decision and draining willpower until the choice is made. Just make the decision as soon as possible.

Identify when a choice doesn't really matter. In the choice of food, does it matter if your dinner is fish or chicken; or if your veggies are corn or peas? Not really.
Also identify times when you have insufficient information to make a deep and meaningful choice. You might have two movies to choose from but haven't heard many reviews of either. It doesn't matter which one you

spend time watching first, you'll likely watch both at some point anyway.

When these occur just make a choice based on a simple mechanic. For the movies you may simply go with the DVD sitting on your left, or alphabetically. For food it's whichever option is closest to you. You may even simply grab the first one you see.

This doesn't mean to allow random chance or proximity dictate what you do. These are simply tools to use when the choices are equal and neither one really matters as you will still be fed and entertained.

Sacrosanct Rules

Create several personal rules that can't be violated. Some examples might be: I avoid soft drinks and alcohol; I eat foods only on this specific list; I train at least once a day; I spend Sunday mornings writing. Keep them as positive as possible, or neutral at the least.

Having created these rules, when faced with a choice of breaking it or not, there is no willpower to spend. The act of creating the rules made the decision and spent the required willpower already. You don't need to do so every time thereafter. Sticking to these rules becomes easy when you have done it for a while.

When starting out it helps to have a penalty for breaking them. This gets you in the habit of following your own rules, or you must sacrifice something important to you. If you are having trouble sticking to these enlist the aid of a friend or life coach to keep you honest. It is easy to set penalties but ignore them if you don't have a monitor or sponsor. After a month you shouldn't need this external check anymore.

The opposite of this, which we should avoid, is to justify a decision with a question. For example, "I ate well yesterday but now I've been offered free cake. Is it OK to have some?"

This question will tap into your WT. Even if you make the decision not to eat the cake, you have drained your willpower, likely a lot. This is where taking precautions helps, see below.

Stick with these rules and they will help make rapid decisions and keep you on track.

Precuations

Think about the common issues that might thwart you during the week and plan your actions ahead of time.

You know a party is coming up on the weekend and they will have cake and alcohol. Think about how they will be offered to you. Make the decision now that when that offer is made, you will politely say "no thanks". There is no need to elaborate. You can also plan to bring your own snacks and drinks such as a muesli bar, some fruit and coconut water. That way you are not going hungry or thirsty while there is so much junk food and unhealthy beverages all around you.

If you are uncomfortable with saying no and leaving it at that, you can embellish it a little. Have a few basic phrases prepared that you can rattle off. Something like "I'm too full from all the lovely food" or "I couldn't possibly fit that in after this feast". These compliment the food on offer and decline politely. This can be helpful if you are just starting out on your healthier choices and don't really want to explain it to everyone you meet.

Expanding this to business or sports, you might be working on a presentation or have some pivotal techniques to rep at the gym. This will take up a lot of your Friday night, which is when you usually go out with your friends. Knowing they will call you to arrange a pickup time, plan to tell them you'll meet up at 10pm after spending time on your work or training. You are then still working, still socialising (just a little bit late) and no willpower has been spent to remain at work or the gym. Going out is then your reward, especially if you manage to finish early.

Think about what will take you off your path before it arrives. Figure out how you will deal with it, and ensure you do that when it crops up. This is like a get-out-of-jail-free card. Having several in your back pocket, you play the card without spending any willpower.

Environmental

Change your surroundings to support you and your goals. If there is no junk food in the house there is no temptation or easy access when you are hungry or emotional. If you have to go to the store to buy the junk food, you probably will just stay at home.

You can also include this in a precaution plan. Anytime you feel like getting junk food, ensure you walk to the shops. That will give you some exercise, but also take up a significant amount of time. If you don't have the time then it's more incentive to stick at home and continue with your schedule, without dipping into your Willpower Tank.

If a dirty house makes you frustrated or anxious then have strategies and goals in place to clean small areas each day. Ensure this covers your friends and social circles as well. Stick with people that have the same or similar goals as you, or at the very least will support you.

If you are managing your own business find people that are doing the same. Lose weight with your loved ones and friends. Find a gym with people motivated to achieve the same results you desire.

Our surroundings should reflect, enhance and nurture our goals. Not having this only forces us to use willpower to continue around the issues.

Your Identity

Think about the type of person you are. I'm the type of person that goes to the gym every day. That is who I am so it takes no willpower to continue to do that. It would actually take willpower to stop going to the gym as doing so would violate my identity.

We connect a pre-existing identity to whatever goal we want. This can be difficult to discover but think about what resonates with you today. If you need any help, coaches of all types are available. A good coach will be able to find something that makes you tick.

Let's use an example. You might be someone that won't settle for suboptimal results in your business. That is part of your identity and takes no willpower to maintain. However you are overweight and have many aches and pains that might distract you from your business.

Tie your goal of eating right and going to the gym with your identity of not settling. You reshape your identity to also be someone that doesn't settle for suboptimal food choices. You won't settle for a gym with anything less than the equipment, instructors and attitude that will support your goals. You won't settle for suboptimal performance in your exercises.

Overweight to Fighting Weight

Now that this is part of your identity, you don't need willpower to do it. Settling is not who you are, and it is easy to remain true to yourself once you identify it.

There are a few things that may be required to reinforce this new identity, and several that require a life coach to solidify. In general, take a deep breath, close your eyes and visualise yourself acting within this new identity. Ensure you are relaxed prior to starting and take five to ten minutes for the exercise. Fully step into yourself at 1, 3 and 12 months from now, one at a time, and embody doing these activities. See what you would see, hear all the sounds and feel how you'll expect to feel. Collect all this sensual data and bring it back to yourself in the now, and watch it absorb into your being. You'll be amazed at how powerful this can be.

<u>Basic Charisma</u>

You may be wondering why I am including a chapter on charisma in a weight loss book. At first glance they are unrelated, but have a think about why you want to lose weight and how it will alter your life.

Apart from the obvious health benefits you will likely feel better about yourself. You will probably spend more time around people and may do things you never thought possible. From my experience being excessively overweight, it is a solitary existence, even when surrounded by family and friends.

Even though I had loved ones and friends to spend time with, I couldn't enjoy every aspect with them. My friends were far fitter than me. They wanted to do outdoor activities, go hiking, bike riding or play sports at the nearby oval. I wasn't physically in a state that could join in. So I withdrew.

Making excuses became a master skill. I still saw my friends but missed out on a lot. As I stated earlier, my social skills weren't that great to begin with. Making new friends was difficult. To avoid disappointment I hardly spoke to new people I met. It took months for me to relax enough and begin opening up to new people. That is not conducive to making friends and required them to stick around an awkward person long enough to establish trust. I hadn't given any reason for them to want to know me, so why would they bother?

Thinking back on how I was, I wonder how I ever kept friends or even convinced my wife to start dating me. But with massive weight loss I found myself able to do more. One of my most exciting days was when I felt comfortable going to the beach and taking off my shirt for a swim. Previously I wanted to hide everything beneath the obfuscating layers of clothing. Now I wanted people to stare at me in admiration rather than disgust.

With a new confidence brought about by a slimmer me, I needed to understand how to interact with people and have awesome experiences. So this chapter is about understanding charisma to break out of your shell and meet new people.

If you already have these skills, that's fantastic. This chapter will simply reinforce what you already know. For those of you like me, this chapter will help bring you socially closer to the person you feel like with your new body.

The few unusual items in the 8 week guide at Step 1, such as smiling in the mirror and enthusiastic greetings, will make more sense after this chapter.

This is not meant as a complete guide to charisma; that will take a few books alone. The following is a crash course in getting started. While the items here can be dropped in at any time, I recommend delving into this in Step 3 Review Habits. The positivity will balance any negative thoughts brought on by that step.

So let's begin at the first encounter.

Making a Good First Impression

When you meet someone for the first time it can be daunting. I'm introverted and have been quite shy in the past; that doesn't mean I can't make killer first impressions. If I allowed excuses I would do what I did at University, which was keep to myself, stay in the corner at the few parties I was invited to and only speak to people I already knew.

I look back and cringe at all the wasted opportunities at meeting someone that could have made an impact on my life. But I avoided them instead because my shyness was a safety net that kept me secluded in fear. Meeting people shouldn't be difficult, and there are a few things we can do to ease the process.

The first step is to understand the mindset. We do not want to go into an interaction with the thought "how can I make them like me?" or "how can I make a great impression?"

Name dropping people you know comes off as trying too hard and not genuine. Flaunting your status can seem like bragging or make them cram up from intimidation. All of this is the wrong frame of mind, and puts pressure on you.

The goal of a first meeting with someone should be to evoke an emotional response, and have the person link that emotion to you. We need to think "how can I have fun with this person?" and "does this person have something awesome about them that will make them great friends?"

This mindset puts focus on fun and finding out more about them, which is exactly the point of making a new friend.

To make a good and lasting first impression you need to instil four things with the other person in the correct order. Doing these out of order will hinder your efforts. For example your motives may be questioned if establishing respect before showing you can be trusted. These are emotions or states that you want the other person to see coming from you.

The emotions are:

- Positivity. Having fun and being uplifted.
- A feeing of Trust
- Respect
- Genuine Interest

Positivity

Starting at the beginning we want to show our positivity. The easiest way to do this is to provide energy into the situation. If you watch Will Smith enter a room as a guest on any talk show, you will see how pumped he makes everyone just by walking in. We can't all have his energy at the flick of a switch, so the baby step is to have a great answer to the first question nearly everyone asks: How are you?

The default answer to this is "Good thanks, and how are you?"

What does that actually do to improve the conversation let alone your positivity or fun? It is a waste of potential. Imagine instead that when asked this simple question you state enthusiastically "I'm fantastic thank you", or "I'm doing awesome".

The important take away here is that you are exuberant and personify the trait you are claiming to be. Saying "I'm awesome" in a monotone does not convey the sense of awesomeness. This must be real to create a shift in attitude. The best way to achieve this is to genuinely feel good about your life. For some of you this might be a challenge but we only need to focus on small changes to make big impacts.

Practice smiling in a mirror so you can see how others will see you. Even record it on your phone and play it back. We want to see a genuine smile. Fake smiles don't touch the eyes and usually the mouth goes left to right. A genuine smile pulls your mouth up and crinkles the eyes. Think about something positive or fun and be willing to laugh at yourself. Be silly in the moment to see what a true smile of yours looks like. You can then re-create that when meeting new people.

Trust

This is mainly done with body language. The two biggest aspects are touching and eye contact. Ensure when you meet someone you shake their hand and make eye contact for a good few seconds. If you feel game you can even give a bro hug to a guy, or air kiss a girl if appropriate. This usually won't fit into a business setting but might be fine at parties. A firm shoulder clasp also does wonders but pick your times.

You don't want people feeling uneasy from inappropriate touching. If you are unsure, either watch how other people in the setting are greeting each other, or stick to the handshake. Make sure you give the person your undivided attention for a few seconds.

When in group situations you need to touch everyone in the room before moving on. This might mean a simple hand shake with eye contact while repeating their name. You can't expect trust without making eye contact, especially when you are speaking.

Reveal your palms to others when speaking. They should be rigid, not floppy. This shows you have nothing to hide. During the conversation reveal something that may be embarrassing to you. Don't try to play it cool or hide awkwardness. Own it. You might be at a party and don't know many people. Admit you are feeling lost at the party and don't know anyone. Say it with a genuine smile and maybe a chuckle. Owning this vulnerability builds trust as you are happy to share yourself with others.

Respect

Respect may be implicit from context. If you are a CEO of your company then respect is usually implied. If respect is forced before establishing trust then people can feel manipulated. The easiest way to gain respect is to lead the conversation. Be comfortable in steering the conversation to topics you are interested in. For example when someone says something interesting you might say "Hold on a second, you just did X, tell me more. What was that like?"

Don't just blow smoke up their butt to get the conversation rolling. It is easily recognised, even if just as an off feeling. Definitely don't fake it. Ensure you make eye contact with everyone in the group for several seconds each as you talk so they feel included. Don't just dart your gaze around the room, lock eyes for 5 seconds then move on. It will greatly increase their interest and help establish respect.

Genuine Interest

Showing interest is fairly easy when we are steering the conversation, but to make others feel at ease with us we need to make a connection. Within in a few minutes of talking about a topic you often find something in common. You know when you have made a connection by them nodding along with you as you speak, and maintaining eye contact. Now is the time to turn it back on them.

You might say something like "I've been talking for a while now. What is your story?" Leave this deliberately vague. If they want to share something they will go right into it. If not they will probably ask "what do you want to know?" Answer with "whatever you are interested in and care about." It is a rare person that won't have anything to say after that.

Remembering Names

During the entire discussion use their name often. Everyone loves to hear their own name as it brings a connection. It shows you are interested in them.

Don't be afraid to get it wrong. If you do, apologise but then make some fun. Ask them a favour to help you not forget. Anytime you do, ask them to slap you in the face. Remember to chuckle and smile. They likely won't slap you but it can be a silly interaction that will make them remember you.

It also helps to personalise a question using their name and asking for their opinion. "Say Trevor, what did you think of that movie?" Have genuine interest in their response.

You can also associate an internal image or emotional link with their name and face. Tie this back to the context you met them in where possible. This way the next time you see them you should be able to remember their name. Use it immediately and you will make them feel special because you took the time to remember them.

As a coach I meet a lot of new people and can easily forget their names. When I greet them I shake their hand, repeat their name, make eye contact and smile. I give them a basic line on what to expect from the night and move on. During the session I repeat their name as much as possible.

Overweight to Fighting Weight

If I've forgotten a name I joke with them, usually telling them I'm horrible with names so just punch me a few times and I'll remember. As it is almost always in pairs or trios everyone laughs and breaks any possible tension. I generally only have to ask no more than three times before I remember reliably.

Answers to Common Questions

A great way to establish some fun is to have unexpected answers to all the questions people ask when making chit chat. We already covered "How are you?" The next questions, especially with new people is "What do you do?" and "Where are you from?"

Answer these questions by telling a little story. Include why you do your job, why you live where you do and what you love about it. A simple answer for what I do is:

"I work in IT but am passionate about writing, life coaching and teaching martial arts."

With this I have provided four avenues for further questions being IT work, writing, coaching and martial arts. They will usually pick one they are interested in to ask further questions. If not, you can elaborate with why you love what you do. Speaking with passion will rub off on them. If they still don't ask many questions, ask an open ended one yourself to get them talking about their passions. Use the one in the genuine interest section above to get started.

Don't be afraid to test your answers on new people at the same event. Mix up your words and see which ones get the best response. For example, I could use the word "writer", "author" or "novelist" to describe that aspect. Changing "life coach" to "health coach" or "personal mentor" will have greater impact on different types of people. Each word evokes a slightly different reaction. Play with them to see what provides the best openings for discussion in that context.

I've also used an interesting way to describe my IT work at a government agency that demands a follow up question. When asked what I do, I answered "I help protect the state's infrastructure from malicious attack." I've also used "I'm the complaints wall."

Both of these are vague and could mean anything. Further questions guide my responses but if I get blank stares, I clarify with a cheeky smile and they usually laugh.

Simple Body Language

How we move our bodies speaks volumes. Filling as little space as possible appears timid. Using a lot of space shows confidence and power. There are a few simple things we can do to improve how people perceive us. The added benefit is that the more we use positive body language, the sooner it alters our mood and mentality to match.

Stance is a big one. The superman pose, legs shoulder width apart with hands on hips, is great at embodying power. Just standing here for a minute builds confidence. Slight adjustments such as taking a step back to angle away makes it less imposing during conversation, especially if you are tall like me.

Fill your area. Use straight arm gestures instead of keeping elbows in tight. Utilise shoulder movement instead of the elbows. Don't be too stiff or too loose, simply relax. Adjust your torso when making sweeping gestures.

Overweight to Fighting Weight

Utilise sound to enhance your speech. Snapping your fingers will not only highlight a point, but will also return focus to you. Commanding attention is a large part of charisma and maintaining the focus of others is huge.

Use this sparingly and for emphasis only. People don't like finger snapping to gain their attention when distracted or uninterested. The finger snap at the key point puts the underscored word into memory, and forces a refocus as people may have missed something important.

All of this builds confidence the longer you use it. This has a profound impact on your mindset and in a very short time you will ease into leading a conversation.

Homework

None of this will help unless you practice. So for the first week create some goals from the guidelines above. We only need little changes to build momentum. This first week will look something like this.

- **Day 1. Be Awesome**. When asked how I am, respond enthusiastically. Words to use include awesome, great, stellar, fantastic, terrific and wonderful. Have a big, genuine smile. Do this all day. Make a mental trigger by thinking about when you usually see people and visualise yourself doing this in the usual setting. Take notes at the end of the day about how it worked and how you felt.

- **Day 2. Introductions.** Go out of your way to introduce yourself and ensure you touch everyone with a handshake. Break people out of their routine. Create a mental trigger from a minute before the interaction as a visual tool then follow it all day. Take notes on how it all went.

- **Day 3. Answer to "Where are you from?"** This should be three to five sentences. Share your values and passions. Leave hooks and open loops for the other person to pick up on. Be enthusiastic. Practice saying it until it's comfortable, then utilise it in the wild. Take notes at the end of the day and see if you need to alter it.

- **Day 4. Answer to "What do you do?"** Again this should be three to five sentences, share your values and passions and use open loops and hooks. Ensure the answer includes why you do it and where it gets you in life. Practice until it is natural and use it in the wild. Take notes at the end of the day and alter as required.

- **Day 5. Eye contact.** Engage in strong eye contact especially when speaking. It is hard to think straight when speaking and looking directly into someone's eyes. Visualise doing it before any interaction and ensure you smile. Take notes on how easy or difficult this was, and why you felt that way.

- **Days 6. Power Stance.** Spend time working on being in a power stance and filling space with your presence. Practice in a mirror first, and then unleash it in the wild. Extra points if you can work in a finger snap at the right moment. Take notes about how you felt and how you think it altered conversations.

- **Day 7. Repeat trouble days.** Your notes after each day will highlight what you need to work on. Do so on day 7 as much as possible to reinforce your problem areas. Update your notes so you can adjust accordingly in the next week.

Further assistance

There are far more avenues with improving charisma and confidence than is within scope for this book. If you want to delve further you can contact me with the details in the final chapter and we can have a chat.

One critical source in gaining this knowledge was Charlie Houpert from Charisma on Command. Check out his YouTube channel and once you see the gold mine of information, consider his Charisma University courses.

<u>Altering Behaviours and Triggers</u>

One of the major factors in why I became so overweight was how I dealt with certain triggers. My default response to frustration, boredom, anger, disappointment and many others was to eat.

I love playing video games and have been known to spend entire weekends with zero sleep playing them. Previously I always had snacks near me so when there was a loading screen I would have something to eat or drink. That was usually junk food.

Understanding this behaviour and recognising the trigger point was critical in stopping it. I don't necessarily need to stop eating during load screens, as long as I am eating the right food. A fruit salad can be a wonderful snack and I still get hungry playing games over long hours. It's the recognition that is key.

If you are already thinking of common triggers for your eating then fantastic, you are half way there. If not, Step 3 Reviewing Habits will help discover the majority.

When looking over your feelings immediately prior to eating in Step 3, we are looking for commonalities. If you notice you reach for food when frustrated you have just recognised a trigger.

Take some time evaluating this data until you are fairly confident you have exhausted the list. It's OK if you miss a few as we will re-evaluate after adjusting the first pass.

With a list of triggers we can move onto adjusting our behaviour towards them.

Avoidance

This is one instance where avoiding the trigger is a good start. For example, assume you get frustrated when people text your phone while you are busy working on a project. The simple way to avoid this is to turn your phone on silent; or not have it in the same room or within earshot.

People do not generally live up to your expectations. They may always be late, might pay back money weeks past the agreed date or a multitude of other little things that bug you. You will have similar traits that annoy other people, it's unavoidable.

But we can manage what we expect of others when we understand how they normally behave.

I have a friend that is always late, let's call him Bob. When saying to meet up at 10am Bob will get in the shower at 9:55am. So while we wait for Bob to be ready, we reach for a snack.

Bob has time management issues with a busy schedule. He wants to spend time with me and our friends but other things take precedence. I know Bob enjoys the time we spend together. Rather than getting triggered when Bob is late, I can manage my expectations.

One option is to work with Bob to alter the start time. While we could lie to Bob and tell him we are starting at 9am, it will only work a few times until Bob catches on. He might also get angry at being lied to.

Another option is to not put Bob in a position where timing is critical. Discuss beforehand if Bob is likely to make it on time and he can decide if it's important enough to schedule in. We can also ensure Bob understands everyone else will be starting at a specific time with or without him. He then knows if he is late he may miss out or must make his own way to the event.

Some things cannot be avoided and in these instances take 30 seconds to think about the situation. Reacting without thinking is where we get in trouble and reach for a snack. We can't immediately alter our automatic reaction to triggers, but we can choose how to behave once they hit.

A trigger of frustration will still make us frustrated, but taking time to think before grabbing a chocolate bar will avoid breaking our energy budget. It will also avoid having to spend willpower.

Breathing

With how critical breathing is to continued life I find it horrifying that we don't use it to its fullest. A deep breath provides more than just oxygen to enrich our blood. Relaxed breathing is necessary to remain calm in frightening or stressful situations.

Diaphragmatic breathing is amazing and will bring you to greater physical awareness and conditioning. I encourage you to do further research into that. The Iceman Wim Hof is a great place to start. Attending his seminar was an experience I'll never forget. For our purposes though, take a few deep breaths whenever triggered by anything.

While taking time to think before reacting, take in a deep breath over four or five seconds. Ensure you fill your diaphragm, you'll recognise it when your stomach fills out. Lifting your shoulders is a sign you are breathing too shallow. Hold your breath for four or five seconds, then relax and allow the air to fall out rather than pushing it out. You should only need to repeat this a few times before you feel calm and relaxed.

Within a short time, breathing should replace your reaction to the trigger, thus avoiding reaching for food or drink. If you are really struggling with this, consider consulting a life coach for advanced techniques.

Mindset Choices

With taking time to breathe and think we can often highlight our current mindset and change it. Before flying off the handle or eating more junk food ask yourself a few questions.

Will this matter tomorrow, next week or next year?
Am I missing something? Are things really how I just perceived them?
Does the other party have all the information I do?
Am I seeing the situation clearly or do I simply want to be right?
Can I get my point across without turning hostile?
Am I taking other people's needs into account?
Will my anger/frustration/boredom/etc help the situation?

Asking these questions after the deep breaths will give you clarity and move you forward, instead of being stuck in the situation and reaching for bad choices.

Again this is a sizable topic that will easily stray beyond the confines of this book. This chapter should provide some insight into where to research if you need more information. You can also contact me for guidance.

Key points

There is a simple order of tasks when triggered to bring you back to normal.

<u>Smile</u>. Even a forced one when triggered can help you return to a happy state.

<u>Breathe</u>. Take at least three deep cleansing breaths.

<u>Think</u>. Ponder the situation and your reaction to it.

<u>Question</u>. Are you reacting to the entire picture? Does it ultimately matter?

With this you can quickly avoid poor behaviour to any trigger. Remember to minimise those triggers in the first place and you will have taken a massive step towards a healthier you.

<u>Beginning Exercise</u>

When starting from the poor physical condition I was in, many exercise programs would have broken me. I could barely do three push-ups before having to stop. So while we slowly alter our meals we need to enhance it with similarly slow progression of exercise. This is why some basic exercise is included in the 8 week guide back in Step 1. They will start building you towards more rigorous exercises without breaking you.

The following is a light start that builds over several levels. There is no set timeframe for changing into the next level as it all depends on your performance. Always strive to push yourself but never at the expense of injury. To start you won't be able to tell the difference between being tired and being in pain that will cause injury if you continue. That will change quickly and after a few months you will know what you can handle without hurting yourself.

There are examples of all of these exercises all across the internet. I'll provide basic instructions at the end of this chapter but I've used exercise names that are found in thousands of videos that are easy to find. I specifically have not included picture or video links as a means to ensure you do some research. Your current physical roadblocks may mean you need very different exercises to blast through. If you think something is too hard then your mind will make it so. If you think it is not yet easy, then your mind will be primed to push through the challenge. Take this book to your sport physiologist (or find one) and they can create something based on your current levels to work towards and beyond this.

Each level will consist of a warm up, the workout section then a warm/cool down and stretch. The time it takes to complete the entire routine will increase as the levels progress. If you are pressed for time reduce the workout section, not the warm up or stretch. The entire point of this is to get your heart rate up and not injure yourself.

Set a relevant goal to do the workout two to four times per week. If you are pushing yourself you should be able to step up a level after one to four weeks.

Level 0 Mission Control

This is the base level to get you used to exercise. When you can complete this entire level without much difficulty in under 12 minutes, move onto Level 1.

<u>Warmup:</u> 30 seconds of star jumps, 30 seconds of squats. Repeat.

<u>Workout:</u> 10 push-ups, 10 crunches, 10 high knees, 10 butt kicks, 10 lunges. Rest for 1 minute. Repeat 3 to 5 times. As you progress, decrease the rest period to 30 seconds in 10 second increments.

<u>Warm down:</u> Jog on the spot for 2 minutes, slowing down every 30 seconds until you are walking. Take long deep breaths during the exercise to control your heart rate.

<u>Stretches:</u> For all of these stretches, go for 10 seconds, rest for 10 seconds, and then stretch again. Groin, hamstring, calves, triceps and pecs.

Level 1 The Launchpad

This is where we begin to test limits. Mental endurance is just as important here. We need to push through the tired barrier and continue even when we want to give up. Move onto Level 2 Lift-off once this

Overweight to Fighting Weight

becomes easy. This entire routine will take just under 40 minutes. For the first week at this level do the workout section 3 times. Then add another round each week until you maintain at the full 5 rounds.

Warmup: 30 seconds of star jumps, 30 seconds of high knees, 30 seconds of burpees, 30 seconds of squats. Start again but with 15 seconds for each exercise. There is no rest until you complete the second time through. It will take 3 minutes.

Workout: This is a timed workout. You will be doing an exercise to the count of 10, then complete the minute with star jumps. If you can't complete 10 of the exercise in a minute then do as much as you can. Switch to the new exercise at each minute mark regardless.

First minute: Push-ups
Second minute: Mountain climbers (10 each leg)
Third minute: Split jumps (10 each leg)
Fourth minute: Burpees
Rest for 90 seconds
Repeat 3 to 5 times.

Warm down: Star jumps for 2 minutes, progressively getting slower every 30 seconds. Take long deep breaths to control your heart rate.

Stretches: For all of these stretches, go for 15 seconds, rest for 10 seconds, and then stretch again.
Groin, hamstring, calves, hips, stomach, triceps and pecs.

Level 2 Lift-off

This level is where we begin to focus on strength. Again we need mental endurance to push our body beyond its current limit. By doing this we push the thresholds further for next time. This will take around 35 minutes. Continue to Level 3 when you can easily hold each position for a minute.

<u>Warm up:</u> 30 seconds of star jumps, 30 seconds of mountain climbers, 30 seconds of slipt jumps, 30 seconds of burpees and 30 seconds of squats. Start again but with 15 seconds for each exercise. Start again but with 10 seconds for each exercise. There is no rest until you complete the third time through. It will take 4 minutes 35 seconds.

If you have a skipping rope, replace this entire warm up with 4 to 5 minutes of skipping. If you get the rope tangled keep jumping while you adjust it. Again YouTube is your friend for detailed instructions but a basic guide is at the end of this chapter.

<u>Workout:</u> We will alternate between a strength exercise and a cardio one. This will be in a 5 minute block between rests.

Forearm plank until failure, aim for 1 minute.
Tuck jumps for 1 minute.
Wall sit until failure, aim for 1 minute.
Star jumps for 1 minute.
Superman hold until failure, aim for 1 minute.
Rest for 90 seconds.

Overweight to Fighting Weight

Burpees for 1 minute.
Side plank until failure, aim for 1 minute.
Hindu push-ups for 1 minute.
One legged squat until failure, aim for 30 seconds.
Mountain climbers for 1 minute.
Rest for 90 seconds.

Crunches for 1 minute.
V-sit until failure, aim for 1 minute.
Lunge for 1 minute.
T-stand Pulse until failure, aim for 1 minute.
Russian twists for 1 minute.
Rest for 90 seconds.

<u>Warm down:</u> Jog on the spot for 2 minutes, slowing down every 30 seconds until you are walking. Inchworm for 1 minute taking the time to do perfect reps. Take long deep breaths to control your heart rate.

<u>Stretches:</u> For all of these stretches, go for 20 seconds, rest for 10 seconds, and then stretch again.
Groin, hamstring, calves, hips, stomach, back, triceps and pecs.

Level 3 Re-entry

This level is basically just intensifying the other levels. Go back to the start and double the reps in the workout section, and double the time in the stretches.

<u>Level 0</u> you'll do 20 of each workout exercise and hold the stretches for 20 seconds each.
<u>Level 1</u> you'll do 20 of each workout in the minute timeframe. Alternatively you reduce the rest period by 30 seconds, or add in another set. Stretches will be for 30 seconds.

<u>Level 2</u> you'll hold the positions for an extra 30 seconds or reduce the rest period by 30 seconds. Stretches will be for 40 seconds.

This keeps you working harder and cycles through the levels to keep it fresh for you. Restarting at easier levels gives you the required rest periods so you don't burn out. Increasing intensity ensures you continue to push yourself. Sweating is the simplest indicator you are working hard enough. If the workouts fail to make you sweat they are inadequate.

Once you cycle through all levels twice you can start mixing in new exercises. There are hundreds available so once you have the pattern, swap in a few new ones to test your capabilities.

Basic Instructions

Most people know the very basic way to perform the common exercises. For those, such as push ups, I'll include key details to ensure they are done in a useful manner that doesn't cause injury. It's better to perform 3 perfect push ups than 30 rushed and poorly executed ones. They are listed alphabetically.

<u>Burpees</u>
Sprawl. Push up. Jump up. A sprawl is placing both hands on the ground and kicking your legs back into a plank. Perform a push up. Jump back to your feet and spring up as high as you can. Do a tuck jump (knees to chest) if able.

<u>Butt Kicks</u>
Run on spot or in laps while kicking your heels up to your butt in unison with each step.

Crunches

Similar to a sit up, however do not curl your back as it puts too much tension on it. Aim to push your chest and chin to the ceiling with a straight back. You only really need to lift your shoulders off the floor a short way.

High Knees

Run on the spot by raising your knees to waist height or higher. Run faster as your ability increases.

Hindu push up

Begin with arms straight and bum in the air. You start in an inverted V with hands and legs as the down strokes and butt as the middle point. Drive your chest down between your hands and scoop you head up at the bottom. Lock arms straight. Your groin should be on the ground while shoulders are up as high as they can. Arms vertical by your side. Hold for a moment, now drive butt back to the starting position. Repeat.

Inchworm

Start standing and place your hands on the floor in front of you. Keep your legs as straight as possible. Walk your hand forward and don't move your legs. Ease into a push up position. You can perform a push up to make this more of a challenge. No inch your feet towards your hands, legs straight until you return to the starting position of feet and hands almost touching. Repeat.

Lunges

Feet shoulder width apart. Take a single step forward and crouch. Keep back straight, head up and hands by your side. Your knee should be just above the floor without touching it. Return to starting position and repeat with opposite leg.

Mountain climbers
Start in a high push up position, i.e. arms straight. Pump your legs one at a time like pistons so that your knee goes a little past your elbow. Your head rises as the knee comes up and lowers as the knee returns. Going slow and perfect is better than fast without the full motion range.

One legged squat
Same as a normal squat however one leg is held straight forward. Lower your standing leg so your butt gets as close to the ground as possible. Take it slow on the downward and upward paths.

Plank, forearm, side
Forearm plank is close to the standard push up position, however you are resting on your forearms instead of your hands. Head up, hips down and back straight.

Side plank has you on a single forearm and leg. Shoulders are perpendicular to the floor. Arm not on the floor reaches straight up while you look to the ceiling. Feet are on top of each other so only one touches the floor. Hold for a few seconds before switching sides and repeating.

Push ups
Key points are to keep your elbows tight to your side so that they just scape your body. Eyes looking forward, not at the floor. Back, bum and legs in straight alignment. Guide your chest to the floor and ensure your chest and chin touchdown at the same time. I do not recommend doing push up from the knees as it's easy to use the wrong muscles. If you have to due to back issues then ensure you are leaning forward so the bulk of your weight is towards your hands and not your knees.

Overweight to Fighting Weight

<u>Russian Twists</u>

Like a V sit though knees are bent and you twist your torso to each side, placing both hands on the ground on the same side before repeating on the opposite side.

<u>Skipping</u>

Aim to only move your wrists when skipping rather than your arms. Jump when the rope touches the ground in front of you. Aim to jump on the balls of your feet with heels close to the ground. Start slow and build up speed as you improve. Maintaining a steady rhythm is the key to success.

<u>Split Jumps</u>

Similar to a lunge but with a jump in between to switch legs. Ensure the knee doesn't touch the ground and jump as high as you can.

<u>Squats</u>

As a minimum you want to squat down so your thighs are parallel to the ground. Back is straight and we don't bend forward. The bum goes backwards as if sitting down. After a few sessions aim to get your bum to the floor. If knee issues prevent the full range of motion, then squats with just your body weight will help improve the condition.

<u>Star Jumps</u>

Start standing with feet shoulder width apart and arms by your side. Jump up enough to spread your legs wide apart and touch your hands together over your head. Jump again and return to the starting position.

<u>Superman hold</u>

Lay flat on the floor stomach down, arms stretched directly in front of you as far as they can. Legs do the same behind. This looks like you are Superman flying. Hold for a few seconds before relaxing. For added intensity instead of relaxing push up on your hands and feet into a plank, hold for a second then lower yourself down. Repeat.

T-Stand Pulse

One foot stays on the floor. Other swings back straight while chest leans forward. Back and raised leg are in perfect alignment forming the top of the T. Solitary leg is the T trunk. Arms can either be at your side or preferably reaching straight forward passed your head.

Tuck Jumps

Jump as high as you can whilst bringing your knees to your chest. Quick jumps are the key, so as soon as your feet touch down you should be jumping again.

V sits

Bum is on the floor. Lean back and raise your legs straight. Keep back and legs at an angle so you embody the shape of a V. Hold for as long as you can. If you get lower back pain during the exercise, then ease off on the angle.

Wall sit

Place your back onto a wall that won't fall over or collapse with pressure applied. Slide down so you are in a squat position ensuring your thighs are parallel with the ground. Remain here for a set time before relaxing. If you press your back into the wall then it will help get through the burn. To increase the intensity and challenge, place a Swiss ball between your legs and squeeze it with your knees.

Stretches

There are many ways to stretch out your muscles, the following are a sample that most people should be capable of with some effort. These can always be built upon and made harder. Always start at a low effort and build up as you progress.

Back
Option 1: Lay flat with arms at your side. Raise your legs straight and place them above your head. The aim is to touch your toes above your head with unbent legs. Breathe out during the exercise and breathe in when returning back to the starting position. Only go as far as you are able. Most people should be able to get their feet in line with their eyes. That is a good start but if you experience pain ease back.

Option 2: Sit down with legs directly in front. Place your right leg over your left so that your right foot is on the floor next to your left knee. Bring your left elbow to the right side of your right knee, looking over your right shoulder. Switch to the other side.

Calves
This works best with a wedge you can stand on however a box will suffice if you have something to grab for balance. The point is to have your toes at an angle higher than your heels with your legs straight. Both legs are stretched simultaneously. Keep your back straight and hips forward. Grabbing something in front of you helps maintain this, even simply placing your hands on the wall. Hold for as long as you can but no more than 2 minutes at a time.

Groin
Sit down with legs directly in front. Spread your legs apart until you feel tightness. Point toes directly up. Lean forward and while looking straight ahead try to get your chin to the ground. Not many people can actually touch the ground with their chin in this stretch, however the attempt helps stretch in the correct locations. Sit back up

and try to place your chin on each knee one at a time while reaching for your toes.

Bring your legs close slightly to ease of the stretch for a few seconds, then attempt to stretch the out further than the first set. Use your hands to help. Repeat the steps before relaxing and shake out your legs prior to standing.

<u>Hamstring</u>
There are more options here than others because if you sit down most of the day then hamstrings need the most work. They impact back and hip flexibility so working here will help several areas.

Option 1: Sit with left leg straight and the right bent so your heel is at your groin. Push up on your hands and move your butt closer to your heel then drop back down. This ensures maximum targeting of the stretch. Lean forward, aiming for your chin to touch your knee (it's OK if it doesn't). Reach for your left toes with your left hand. Keep your left toes pointed to the roof. Switch legs.

Option 2: Stand feet shoulder width apart. Bend straight down trying to put your head between your legs. Ensure legs remain straight. If they bend at the knees ease back until you can keep them straight. As you progress move your legs closer together and eventually put your nose on your shins while grabbing behind your knees.

Option 3: Stand in a lunge position but relaxed on the lower leg, knee on the ground. Sit up straight. Roll your hips forward as if you are attempting to point your groin to the roof. Hold this position

Overweight to Fighting Weight

<u>Hips</u>

Sit down with your left knee raised, foot on the floor. Place your right foot on your left thigh, heel as close to your hip as possible. Drop your right knee towards the floor and hold for the duration. If you feel knee pain back it off a little. Switch legs.

<u>Pecs</u>

You require a vertical structure such as a doorframe for this. Place your palm on the doorframe and step away far enough so your arm is straight. Gently push your shoulder forward and rotate your opposite shoulder away. Switch arms.

<u>Stomach</u>

Lay flat on your stomach, place hands on the ground and push up keeping your hips touching the floor. Arms should be straight and head held high. Concentrate on pushing hips down and head back.

<u>Triceps</u>

Stand up straight. Place you hand on your spine near your neck. Use your other hand to gently push down on your elbow so that your hand travels lower down your back. Stop if there is pain. Change arms.

Further Steps

Work on adding things like handstands, cartwheels, forward rolls, bear crawls, alligator walks and scorpion hops to your warm ups. Find new stretches to target similar areas to switch in and avoid stagnation.

The ability to complete Level 0 Mission Control once should give you the confidence to start any sport with the knowledge you can do what they require from beginners.

Exercise must evolve or you will become bored and stop doing it. It's OK to slow down for a few weeks, but never stop. Even with injuries there should be something you can still do, just check with the doctors and rehab specialists first.

Combined with the food management above, these exercises will catapult your weight loss and build your strength. The confidence gained from ticking off goals and maintaining motivation will spill over into all aspects of your life. Your updated charisma skills will have you meeting new friends. Utilising everything in this book to its fullest will enable you to tackle whatever life throws your way.

This is just the beginning.

<u>Summary</u>

There is a lot of information above, so this chapter lists the condensed version for quick reference.

<u>Step 1.</u> The 8 Week Guide.
Slowly add health choices to existing meals, increase exercise and begin improving social interactions.

<u>Understand Nutrition Labels.</u>
Review the ingredients then check the nutrient section for carbs, fats, proteins etc. Make educated choices for healthier food.

<u>Step 2.</u> Energy Budget.
Figure out your energy budget and stick to it. Set your own limits and avoid excuses or justifying poor choices.

<u>Step 3.</u> Review Habits.
Note down what you eat, when and your feelings at the time of eating.

Delve into the Charisma section, take time to write everything you are grateful for and focus on positive aspects of your day during discussions.

<u>Step 4.</u> The Elimination Round.
Remove a poor food or drink choice as identified in Step 3 each month for three months.

<u>Step 5.</u> Moderation.
Spend a month to slowly add the removed food back, but in moderation. This is a testing phase to ensure you can enjoy a chocolate bar every once in a while and not let it take over. Remove it immediately if it begins to take hold again.

After several months of going back and forth between steps 4 and 5 you can stop counting kilojoules and simply make healthy choices.

<u>Step 6.</u> **The Ultimate Push.**

Strict meal plan with increased exercise to drop the last stubborn kilograms. No more than twice a year and at least 6 months apart. Navigate a month of difficulty and then stabilise on the other side.

Mental Endurance.

To change the mental aspects of weight loss you need a framework to build upon. Understanding yourself allows insight into improving any aspect that is counterproductive to achieving your goals.

<u>Understanding Motivation</u> means to strive to re-attain moments of high motivation and recognising the signs of heading down the low path.

<u>Setting appropriate Goals</u> is critical to keep you focused and works hand-in-hand with managing motivation.

<u>Charisma</u> and understanding social interactions will increase personal happiness and can change your mindset, getting you out of the funk generally associated with massive weight gain.

<u>Managing your Willpower</u> will ensure you can stick to your goals, stay motivated, keep within your energy budget and get things done.

<u>Breaking through Plateaus</u> will be possible once the above is adhered to and mastered.

<u>Recognising and Managing Triggers</u> will launch you into mastery over yourself, and demolish all barriers that stand in your way.

Physical Activity

<u>Exercise</u> increases progress in stages. Start with the basics and push harder in increments. Ensure fresh exercises are switched in to keep stagnation at bay.

Overweight to Fighting Weight

Resources
Use this example table to track your daily intake during Step 2 Energy Budget and Step 3 Review Habits.

Intake	Oats 30g
Time	7am
Kj	477
Protein	3.6g
Fat	2.6g
Carbs	16.8g
Sugars	0.4g
Fibre	3.8g
Sodium	<5mg
Thoughts & Feelings	Sleepy, hungry

You can make this as complicated or as simple as you wish. Using a spreadsheet application such as MS Excel you can add in calculations for number of serves, auto-add totals, create pull-down menus for commonly eaten foods that auto-fills the data etc. If you want something like that and are not yet a guru at spreadsheets, please send me a message and I'll whip something up for you.

The following websites are great resources for further study, to assist in calculations, give tips or just general knowledge to support you.

Charisma on Command
Great advice on social interactions and methods to improve the quality of your conversations and friendships. The Charisma University helped me a lot and I highly recommend it.

<u>Fitness Blender.</u>
Go to the section for Free Workout Videos. Great search tool for exercise routines at various levels. Videos and transcript detail the steps and you can work along with them.

<u>www.8700.com.au</u>
Great for energy budget calculation, food search, health tips and more.

<u>Webcalcsoultions.com</u>
They have a great calculator in their Fitness section for figuring out your percentage of body fat. Use the US Navy Method and ignore BMI completely.

There are many great sites to help develop everything discussed to greater heights. A Life Coach will propel you even higher. Contact me for more information.

Links and Contact Details

Keep this book somewhere in easy reach so you can refer back often. You'll see remarkable results in a matter of months but keep it going. I'm still adjusting things in my own training and food intake, and continue to improve.

I still enjoy some junk food in moderation. Restricting yourself fully will only break your willpower and motivation. If you stray too far you can easily go back a few steps to bring everything back in check. As stated earlier, this is not a diet book but a structured system to manage your weight, exercise and energy levels. If you utilise all the skills and knowledge contained within then you'll achieve your goals.

If you are struggling with any aspect of this, there are tools to help break habits and make new associations with undesired treats. Contact me to discuss my coaching services and how I can assist you realise your dreams.

I would love to see your before and after pics. You can get in contact with me via the avenues below.

Website: www.ajwatson.com.au
Coaching Site: www.ajcoaching.com.au
Facebook: www.facebook.com/aj.watson.author
Twitter: www.twitter.com/AJWatson_
Email: ajw@ajwatson.com.au

Finally you can join the community on my Patreon page to get more insights, and gain access to all of my novels and other books. This is a "DVD extras" site for my writing and I'd love to see you there.

Patreon: www.patreon.com/AJWatson

AJ Watson

I wish you nothing but the best and hope to hear from you soon. Enjoy your new healthy and active body. You deserve it.

AJ Watson.

<u>About AJ Watson</u>

AJ Watson (Tony to his friends) lives with his wife Barbara in the great state of Victoria, Australia.

AJ is a certified Life Coach and continues to expand his skills to assist others not only duplicate his successes but to clear any mental barriers people place upon themselves.

Tony has obtained a Bachelor of Computing and although he has a love of technology, he can't help dreaming of worlds with vicious creatures and powerful metaphysics. He uses this imagination to write sci fi/fantasy novels.

Tony is an experienced martial artist competitor and instructor, having won multiple national gold medals and assisting others to do the same.

In his spare time, among other things, Tony dabbles in computer graphics and GMs many role play games with his family and friends.

Also by AJ Watson

The Gatekeeper Trilogy
Embark on a journey with Velus, a former street urchin from a primitive planet, as he is thrust into a universe beyond his understanding. The Void War has consumed over a dozen civilisations and threatens far more, with an ancient evil determined to escape their eternal prison. Powerful elemental energies are flung from both sides, sowing chaos in its wake. The fate of the galaxy is in the hands of Velus and his assortment of allies from multiple worlds. Can he confront his destiny

and survive; or will the forces overwhelm and crush it? Or perhaps there is a third choice?

Void War: The Gatekeeper Trilogy begins with **The Elemental Progeny**, continues in **The Shroud of the Gods** and concludes with **The Keeper of Sin**. Available now at major online book retailers.

Inquisitor Qyr Chronicles

Do you like fantasy with a sprinkle of sci fi? **Arson's Canvas** will ignite your imagination, touring a rich world filled with intrigue and running on elemental power.

Qyr is an Inquisitor for The Trust, the law enforcement agency of planet Volyce. He loves his job investigating serious crimes in a town not far removed from the frontier status during the rush for mining ore. One thing he loves more than his job is his privacy. However that is threatened when a murderer destroys a monastery in a blast of fire only the greatest practitioners of the elements could muster.

The wanton destruction exposes secrets of several powerful organisations as Qyr conducts his inquisition; secrets that shake the foundation of even The Trust itself.

That pales to the personal conflict for the Inquisitor. His extensive history is filled with details best left to the past. Balancing between privacy and duty, Qyr must learn the secrets of his birth before they attack the life he has built.

Who can he trust with enemies encroaching on all sides, even among those seeming to help?

Join Inquisitor Qyr as he Chronicles his journey so he can understand a choice that will impact millions.

Coming Early 2018.

Thank you and best wishes.